GOLF YOURSELF TO LIFE

Why and how to get started in
the greatest sport on the planet

Andrew Cullen, PGA Professional

Rethink

First published in Great Britain in 2021
by Rethink Press (www.rethinkpress.com)

Disclaimer

The use of any information in this book, including any suggested exercise, is solely at the reader's own risk. You should always seek medical advice before undertaking any exercise or starting an exercise program. Neither Rethink Press nor the author can be held liable or responsible in respect of any and all injuries, losses, damages, expense, or other adverse effects incurred while undertaking any of the exercise or other activities described in this book.

Cover image © www.pexels.com

Picture credits: Photographs by Foto Digital Stotzer AG; Figure 2 Shutterstock|amanemark; Figure 3 Shutterstock|VAZZEN; Figure 4 Shutterstock|Colin Hayes; Figure 19 Jeremy Duncan; Figure 20 Jeremy Duncan

CONTENTS

To my parents, Peter and Sydena,
both golf fanatics, who brought
me up into a life of golf

To my partner, Gila, a life fanatic,
who brought me to life

FOREWORD

It is said that golf is a game for a lifetime – you can play from eight to eighty years old. They also say you need this long to learn how to play because it's so difficult! First and foremost, Andrew is a lifelong golfer. Born and growing up in Scotland probably means that the game of golf is in his DNA, just as playing in wind and rain is – in fact, like all Scots Andrew positively smiles (or is it a grimace?) when the trees are doing press-ups.

I first met Andrew when I was coaching in Switzerland, where he has plied his trade for the last two decades. Although busy himself as a coach, he came to me to help him improve his game as a golfer, as he had a dream and vision of one day playing in some Senior Tour events, such as the Senior British Open. This coaching journey with me led him to join our Winter Elite Program in Australia, where he was plunged into a group of young elite players who aspired to play on Tour or were already playing on Tour. The physical program was led by the then leading physio trainer on Tour, the late (and great) Ramsay MacMaster. The memory of Andrew chugging along on a beach at 7am in the morning, doing beetle crawls and bunny jumps up and down sandhills, going shoulder to shoulder with players twenty years his junior at the time, will always be etched into my memory. In fact, when it came to core stability and 'the plank', Andrew often left the young wannabees in shame!

I think this shows Andrew's dedication to not only his game, but to the game itself. He has travelled the globe, investing his time and money in order to understand, and consequently coach, this difficult game better.

I say that being an Elite Coach is not about coaching 'elite players' – it's about coaching any level of player in an elite way. Of course, the coaches standing on the range behind the world's best players get the most adulation. But is coaching a mega gifted player like Rory McIlroy or Dustin Johnson more challenging than coaching a 65-year-old with a hip replacement who has never played before? Andrew is definitely an Elite Coach, with his ability to simplify this challenging game and assist his students in making consistent small steps of progress, firing their enthusiasm and enjoyment of the game.

Golf is a wonderful game as it mirrors life – good times, difficult times, bad luck, and good luck, in a constantly changing environment. It's often cited as the number one character-building sport. I certainly believe so. In this book *Golf Yourself to Life,* Andrew's mission is to popularise golf – making it more fun, flexible and accessible. To broadcast the message of physical, mental and social benefits, and present golf in a more entertaining way.

Andrew has encapsulated almost half a century of golfing memories, rich experiences and his perceptions of these experiences and then delivered them in an entertaining way. It is a wonderful, easy to read book that delivers excellent coaching messages through its stories and anecdotes to assist the club golfer to play better, enjoy the game more and become a lifelong fan of golf.

In a nutshell, it is a great fusion of wise advice delivered through rich and entertaining stories. Enjoy the read – I certainly did.

Jonathan Wallett

European Tour Coach and Academy Director –
Elite Coaching Golf Academy

INTRODUCTION

Life is supposed to be fun.[1] For young humans, and many animals, play is an important part of life. They actively seek to be entertained in a variety of ways, learn from their curiosity, explore their immediate outdoor environment, adapt to challenges, and seek pleasure until they're tired or thirsty or hungry. Who says it has to stop? Why do age or life circumstances have to put an end to the fun, curiosity, learning and challenges? Vibrancy, regardless of age, is the key to living life to the fullest, both at work and at play. To maintain our physical, mental and spiritual well-being, we need to find something that stimulates our vibrancy and curiosity, engages us in its fun and challenge, and puts us in touch with nature. For me, and 60 million others on the planet – young, old and all in between – that something is golf.

Engaging escapism

Let's look beyond the mostly 'fake news' that is often levelled against golf: that it's too hard to learn, too expensive, takes too much time, is only for old people, is elitist, has too many rules and is not a sport for modern times. Most people who can walk, see and throw a ball can potentially play golf. There are thousands of golf facilities worldwide – courses and driving ranges – open to all, where you can start to play at minimal expense. The flexibility to hit a few balls on a driving range or play on pitch-and-putt, 9-hole or 18-hole courses means you can spend as little or as much time as you like playing the sport. I teach kids from six years old to adults over eighty years old, from all ethnicities and walks of life – no barriers there. Every sport, and every society, has rules. As long as they are simple, logical, fair, and are designed and applied to give equal opportunity to everyone involved, rules are a positive creation. And as a sport for modern times, golf has never been so relevant – it takes you outdoors in nature, away from polluted areas, is a switch-off from the stresses of working life, offers physical and mental exercise at a level attainable for everyone, and provides social contact with like-minded people in a challenging, sporting and varied natural environment. If this sport were just invented today, it would be the new boom activity! So, if you're lacking vibrancy, if you feel the need for more activity, more contact with nature, more challenge, new friends, and to de-stress on a regular basis and have more fun, then I seriously recommend that you golf yourself to life.

The aims of this book are to:

1. Get you curious enough to have a go

2. Explain in a simple, logical, enjoyable and modern way the technical and mental skills required to play this great game

I'd love you to experience some of the joy, places, people and events that golf has given me and the millions of others who play and relish this game. It has been my life – and a very good one. In this book and supporting online material, I will present everything you need to get started on your golfing journey, in a fun way.

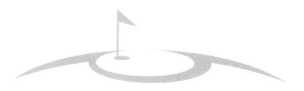

CHAPTER 1

Why Golfers Play Golf

It was a fine summer's day. A light breeze was blowing from the sea. The tide had turned. Some larks were playing and twittering high above our heads in the cloudless, deep-blue sky. The long, fine fescue grass neighbouring the immaculately cut fairways was swirling and whispering mischievously in the breeze like a siren beckoning the golfer's ball to stray in and get lost. There was only myself and a new client on the narrow practice strip at Panmure Golf Club. My client was a nervous type and spoke with a mild stutter. I don't remember his name, but I'll never forget him. I showed him the basics of grip, posture and the critical power move: how to coil the body powerfully on the backswing. After several unsuccessful swipes at the ball came the critical eye-to-ball coordination. Thwack! The ball took off like a rocket, whizzing through the air and silencing the hitherto unperturbed larks. 'Oh m... m... my, I never shit a hot like that before!'

This magical spoonerism marked a significant moment in my career. It was everything that a golf coach could wish for: fun, success, seeing the joy on the face of the golfer, the beautiful setting, and the warm glow as the link between coach and student harmonises and manifests in poetic, synchronised movement and the beautiful flight of a little white ball. It was a realisation that, 'This is what I'm here for.'

I was always a lousy liar. If I ever told a 'little porky' or tried to hide the truth or give an over-diplomatic response, I'd turn red or I'd sound completely unconvincing. Too often, I tried to give what I thought would be the correct reply in the circumstance rather than just telling the truth. A few years ago, I read *How To Be Happy* by Michael Anthony, which suggested one should recite this mantra daily in front of the mirror: 'I am always truthful, positive and helping others.'[2] I did so and discarded any notion of lying to this day. It is very liberating. Therefore, in this book you'll get no lying and no bullshit from me. Instead, you'll get a lot of positivity, which I find is a prerequisite for success in anything.

My reason for writing this book is to introduce you to, and help you enjoy, the great game of golf. In this book, I share the golden nuggets of what I've learned over the past 50 years of playing golf and 30 years of teaching golf. What I know works, particularly for those just starting out.

I come from a family of avid golfers. In 2011, my father was dying from the effects of years of overindulging in the products of his profession – whisky. My last conversation with him was at the Astley Ainslie Hospital in Edinburgh, in 'the deadbeats' ward, as he liked to call it. Nobody ever came out of that ward alive, and most of the patients there were so sick they couldn't even converse with my father, so he found it a lonely place. We chatted about which golf courses he had loved to play the most around Aberdeen where he'd been brought up, sharing fond memories of the classic seaside links courses at Royal Aberdeen, Murcar and Cruden Bay. At the end of my visit, he said, 'I always played my best golf with Wilson golf clubs. Do you think you could get me a set?' I don't know what struck me most: the absurdity of my father thinking he'd ever play golf again when every organ in his body was gradually giving up – he could barely stand up let alone walk or swing a golf club – or how the effects of the strong painkilling drugs he was on kept him unaware of his predicament. Or maybe it was the astonishing devotion to golf that fuelled his belief that one day he would return to the sacred golfing links. I answered, 'Sure'. (This was before I started saying my daily 'be truthful' mantra!) On reflection, his request for a new set of clubs was born out of true dedication to a sport that he was deeply involved in his whole life. I hope my deathbed reflections are less fanatical and more profound but invoked by the same passion and devotion.

My family often played golf together as a three-generation group (or 'flight', as they like to call it in Europe – 'tee-time' in the UK or US). This included: my grandfather, 'Pop' – handicap 12; my grandmother, 'Nana' – handicap 28; my mother – handicap 6; my father – handicap 4; and myself – handicap 3.[3] From our golf swing characteristics, you could never tell we were a family. Pop's swing was slow and deliberate to the top of the swing, like he was loading a catapult, and then he'd smash the club down steeply, sending the ball off barely above head height, with it spending more time running along the ground than it ever did in the air. Effective, but not pretty. Nana was barely 5 foot tall and a slip of a woman, and her club seemed to have more control of her than she had of it. At a painfully tortoise-like pace, the club would make its way up and around her head; a long pause was followed by a ballerina-esque curtsy and 'butterfly-net' catching motion before the club would descend, largely of its own accord, and remarkably, it would somehow make contact with the ball, which popped forwards as if shocked by my Nana's club-wielding efforts. My father's swing was like his temper – fast and furious. In fact, it was so short and fast that I never successfully analysed 'the Blur'. It only ever got slower and decipherable after my father had several whiskies, but then 'the Blur' took on a different meaning. My mother's swing is no technical masterpiece; she rarely practises. But it has rhythm and repeatability and that made her the most consistent and successful of all of us – four-time Ladies Club Champion at Turnhouse Golf Club in Edinburgh. My swing was a mix of all the above, thankfully without the ballerina or butterfly catching attributes. It was also fated with variable results. But I could putt (think mini golf). I could really putt! So could my Pop. And so I learned from a young age – I started to play when I was three years old – that there were many ways to play this game: different swings, different temperaments, different rhythms, all of which could send the ball in its desired direction. And I learned that a great putter was a match for anyone!

I turned professional in 1988 after completing an honours degree in Geography from Glasgow University. My three-year apprenticeship was spent at two of the most prestigious – and, at the time, men-only – clubs in Edinburgh: the Royal Burgess Golfing Society and the Bruntsfield Links Golfing Society. Particularly at the latter, I realised that golf was helping to keep its ageing membership alive: playing 18 holes has some physical challenge involved – especially at Bruntsfield, where hole 17 has a considerable ascent from the fairway to the green – or 'thrombosis hill', as my Pop used to call it. And the social activity, both on the course and in the bar, was, particularly for the widowed men, a great source of joy, comfort and belonging. I spent many days popping the club flag up at half-mast as another old boy kicked it, but the post-funeral celebrations – and they were often genuinely celebrations of the life of a golfing companion – were spent at the club in memory and honour of the deceased, and naturally included a few pink gins or good malt whiskies!

My second job as a head professional was at Newquay Golf Club in Cornwall. For the first time, I was working with low-handicap players in a successful team environment. Through my Professional Golfers' Association (PGA) training, hundreds of hours of further education, endless study of golfing books and technique videos, and increasing experience, I was becoming a proficient teacher. Thankfully, I am also blessed with my mother's patience – to my mind, a prerequisite for a teacher of any discipline. Working with good players and their nuances and fine-tuning requirements was a great eye-opener for me. I taught five County Champions in my seven years in Cornwall: four men and one woman. They could all play the game well before they came to see me – the basic throwing motion, body control and coordination that we will discuss in the next few chapters of this book were already there – but each had their strengths and weaknesses. So, my approach was always to identify what was working well first, before I looked at what was not working well. On many occasions the solution through this approach was easy to find and a simple one: a ball position tweak here, or a grip tweak there. When so many good moves are already installed, one little change can often start a chain of motion which radically improves the performance. Trying to teach them a certain swing method or style could have been, as I found out earlier in my career, counterproductive or at best a slow process to get better results. Unnatural movement could also cause new stresses and strains on the body. So I strived to identify what worked, watched what the ball was doing and adapted as necessary. Everybody and every golf swing are unique.

I moved to Switzerland in 2003. Golf in mainland Europe is refreshingly more mixed than it was in my Edinburgh experiences. Mixed tournaments are commonplace at the clubs in Switzerland. It was a format largely unheard of in my time in Scotland, apart from the odd man-woman partner tournament – or 'mixed foursomes', as it's officially known. My father called it the 'mixed gruesomes' as it was often the source of arguments or day-long silences when blame for one poor shot rapidly deteriorated into a multiplicity of character assassinations. In later years, my mother only played 'mixed gruesomes' with one of her friends' husbands in a much more convivial and successful golfing partnership. 'Finding your happy' on the golf course, as I have learned both through her and in recent years through meditation, is a critical piece of the golfing jigsaw.

A great deal of my teaching time in Switzerland has been spent with beginners: young, old and everyone in between. Many students, and I really mean many, I could have easily classed in the 'no talent/ hope' category on Day One of the learning process. But I have been proved wrong so many times by this category that it no longer exists – particularly by older people who had little or no previous sporting experience but who have gone on to pass their playing tests,* gained tournament experience and an official handicap, and above all now enjoy their time in the golfing environment. At some point, and the time it takes to learn is different for everybody, there comes a 'click', an 'AHA!' moment, or whatever you wish to call it, and things start to work. The natural-based positions and movements that I have tried to install from the beginning, combined with eye-to-ball coordination and a mind-body link, slowly synergise, and bingo! – the stupid little white ball that the Scots for some reason made so small is propelled

---

* In mainland Europe, golfers need to pass two tests to play on the golf course: a theory test – Rules and Etiquette – and a playing test called the 'Platzreife' (literally translated as 'course ripe'). These tests bring beginners up to speed on safety, looking after the golf course, pace of play, and playing to a standard where they, and everyone else on the course, can enjoy their game.

at life-threatening speed through the air to the desired (and sometimes undesired) target. What a great feeling. You'll get it… if you continue reading and practise a little.

It's because my customers 'got it', and because we share this sport, whatever your age or gender, whether you're competitive or not, talented or not, super healthy or not, playing alone or playing with family or friends or people you've never met before, in many beautiful locations around the world, that I write this book. I would like you to try it and experience some of the great things that golf has added to my life. And I want you to struggle less than I ever did to learn it. This game can be complicated if you make it so. From my experience as a teacher with all the modern equipment and knowledge available to us, to best understand through biomechanics how the body can swing the golf club powerfully, efficiently and injury-free, and knowing how to train the mind to act on all the information we receive as we practise, play and prepare to take on the golf course – I believe I can introduce you, at your own pace, in a simple way, to this great game. I haven't created or invented any of this. I am merely the filter and your guide. There's a lot of information out there – some great, some not so great – and I'm just delivering a simplified version in a way that I know works. And I want you to have fun in the process; that's why we 'play' golf.

Golf's pain points

'The recreational golf experience has several pain points that serve as multiple barriers to entry for new audiences. The main ones are:

- *Too hard to learn*
- *Too expensive*
- *Takes too much time*
- *Doesn't align with contemporary social lifestyles*
- *Has an image problem of being stuffy and elitist*
- *Intimidating and complicated'* [4]

Golf participation in many countries is decreasing, and this is another of my drivers for writing this book. It saddens me, and I'd love to reverse the trend knowing how much this great sport can offer. But I also empathise with many of the perceptions in the quote above.

It's a rich old man's sport

It definitely was. And golf has taken a long time to rid itself (particularly in the UK) of this image. My former club in Edinburgh, Bruntsfield, only opened its doors to women members in 2018. It took a young, super-fit, mixed-race kid who changed the game at the top level during the 1990s and 2000s to dispel the old belief that golf is just a game for rich, old men. Thanks, Tiger. His continued golfing success, now into the 2020s, has catalysed many people of all age groups to get involved in this great game.

'It's too expensive' – There have always been artisan clubs, but indeed the high cost of club joining fees and annual subscriptions restricted participation from people in lower socio-economic classes. One of the positive aspects of participant decline is that many clubs have abolished joining fees and are getting more creative in how they accept subscription payments to woo more established and beginner golfers. Where I teach in Germany, we have a 6-month membership for beginners including lessons with the pro, and a reduced-price first year 'trial' membership. In addition, increasingly ubiquitous driving ranges allow non-golfers an easy, no-obligation way to try golf for a few dollars.

It takes too much time

This is a massive theme. For two or three players, it's possible to complete an 18-hole course in 3 to 3 1/2 hours and a 9-hole course in less than 2 hours. The game, purely through the player's lack of knowledge and sometimes a bit of arrogance, is taking too long to play, with 18 holes in 4 1/2 to 5 hours now accepted. Awful. Changes to the rules from the governing bodies in 2019 have encouraged good playing tempo, and hopefully players will endorse them. I am a big fan of 9-hole courses, innovative driving ranges and quality pitch-and-putt facilities. They provide 1 to 2 hours of intensive, fun golf. I am also an advocate of 'no delay' playing – or, as I like to call it, 'no faffing golf' – which we'll cover in Chapter 9. There are so many demands on our time in modern life that when we get a chance to escape with our new sport, it should be a frustration-free, fun, engaging time.

It's too difficult

Apparently, pole-vaulting and golf are two of the most difficult sports on the planet. I can't confirm or deny that statement as I'm scared of heights, and I am sure many other sports would challenge that statement, but what would life be without challenges? I agree that golf is tough – it's three tasks in a single action: create as much speed in the club as possible, connect with a ball the size of a lime that's lying on the ground waiting for you, and send it in the right direction. And if you listen to the well-meaning but frequently disastrous advice from amateur hacks on the driving range, it'll get tougher! But don't fret, just keep reading. I'll keep it simple.

Why the people I teach play golf

In golfers' own words

Obviously, I believe the 'gains' outweigh the 'pains', but I want you to hear it from established golfers as well as from me. In 2018, I sent a questionnaire to all 264 clients on my email list to get their feedback on why they play golf. I asked the following questions:

1. Why did you start playing golf?

2. What do you enjoy most about golf?

3. What do you find most frustrating about golf?

4. How would you recommend golf to non-golfers?

The responses to the first question showed that most golfers are intro-duced to golf by friends or family who already played. Therein lies a big problem for increasing participation: if you don't know anyone who plays golf, you are unlikely to take up the sport, particularly if you've only been exposed to the pain points. So let Hermann, Christine, Katrine, Urs and selected others who responded to my questionnaire – and Erika and Eva, who share their stories of how they started – be the friends who help you understand the fascination and joy that this sport can bring.

1. Why did you start playing golf?

Hermann H: The main reason I started was because I wanted to play a sport that was still possible to play when I got older. Also, my friends had started to play, and I wanted something that got me outside in the fresh air and kept me healthy.

Daniel G: I experienced golf for the first time thirty years ago and decided I would start when my kids grew up. When I could no longer play football and tennis, I took up golf.

The fascination of the sport for me is to be in nature, doing physical activity and discovering new places, and that also motivates me. I have been playing for four years and I am looking forward to the next twenty-five years!

Madeleine R: I played regular tournament tennis from ages twenty-six to fifty-six. The team then split up, and thereafter tennis was no longer fun for me. In tennis, you need to have a partner. In golf, that is not so. One can also play golf to an older age than tennis as it's not so hard on the joints! And so, I began to play golf at fifty-six years old.

2. What do you enjoy most about golf?

Michel M: Golf combines three elements which I much enjoy: the beauty of nature, albeit somewhat adapted to the sport; the sport itself, with the variety of challenges and its wonderful effect on my general health (physical and mental); and the chance to enjoy the company of either family and friends or complete strangers.

Walter B: I can play alone, relaxed, early in the morning, or with colleagues – mostly like-minded, friendly old men like myself, or competitively in a tournament where everybody can play at their own level. I love to be outdoors, smell the grass and watch the birds, and finish the round with a glass of wine!

Matthias S: That old and young, man and woman, big and small, good-handicap and less-good-handicap players can play together and have a fun round of golf.

3. What for you is the most frustrating thing about golf?

Michel M: Frustration? Largely a question of attitude. It's a game one should not take too seriously. Still, after a nice shot, I feel that now I got it, only to blow the next one; that's frustrating!

Peter S: When the ball doesn't do as I planned!

Wayne M: Endless paralysis by analysis on the terrace by one and all trying to justify that actually they can play much better golf were it not for bad luck, the tree in the way, flight partner coughing, etc, etc.

Christine M: No frustration, really. Ups and downs for sure, but that helps motivate me to get better.

4. How would you recommend golf to non-golfers?

Christoph H: It's never boring, outside in the fresh air, sporty without being exhausting, variable, demanding, worthwhile.

Irene V: It's a sport for life. It will improve your health because it requires concentration, fitness and coordination. One can play it alone, with family, with friends, or with strangers and all over the world. One is always in beautiful places with like-minded people, and golfers are generally very likeable people.

Herbert L: The best start is with a good teacher. Then, find a partner who is a good and serious golfer from whom you can learn a lot through watching and imitating. They will also help you with etiquette and to get a feel for 'the spirit of the game'.

Erika and Eva's stories

'WOW! SHIT! WHAT A SHOT!' – ERIKA J

In August 2005, my husband took part in a one-week golf taster course in Bad Bellingen, in South Germany. Very quickly, he was infected by the golf virus. Full of enthusiasm, he and his friends played round after round of golf even in the cold wintertime. As I now know, there is no bad weather on a golf course, only inadequate clothing.

During this time, I took part in some social events at the golf club, and I pedalled up the 'Frickberg' on my bike in spring, drank something with the many nice people at the club and rode home again. They often asked me why I didn't want to take up golf, too. But this was not an option for me; perhaps later, once I had retired. And every time I saw some of the rather big-bellied golfers, I thought: 'Well, getting in the golf cart, driving a few metres, swinging the golf club a little bit from time to time, then starting the same procedure again. And this is called a sport? Not really, not in all honesty. Can't be.'

To prove to the people at the club that golf was not for me, I took part in a one-week golf taster course in Bad Bellingen at the end of April 2006. At the start, my sceptical attitude was not exactly appreciated by the golf pro and my remarks during the course were not always very nice. And then it suddenly happened: the beginner's luck. I hit a really big shot and exclaimed, 'Wow! Shit! What a shot!' The golf pro looked scornfully at me and said, 'Such an expression does not belong on a golf course. On a tennis court, perhaps. But not on a golf course.' Heavens, where was I? I pulled myself together for the next swing and didn't say anything, although I nearly burst. Then the golf pro said again, 'Keep your emotions under control.' How stuffy. And then I had to learn the rules and etiquette – old-fashioned to the point of being impossible.

However, my husband still claims today that I came home on the Thursday evening of this trial week and said, 'On Saturday, we'll go shopping for golf equipment,' which we did. Fortunately, I was able to play on the golf course on the Frickberg, in the company of my husband, with the German licence I then had. We played golf on Saturday, Sunday and Monday – or at least I tried to. On Tuesday morning, on the way to the office, I thought about what kind of work would be waiting for me... and at that moment I realised that I hadn't thought about my work for the last three days – a completely new experience!

Happily, I too have been infected by the golf virus. The following summer, we booked golf holidays in Tirol, Austria. We played in the same flight with many lovely people. Some of them were quite old, and this was another aspect of golf that impressed me. Which other hobby can you enjoy till old age, being out in the fresh air for hours and afterwards drinking and eating something delicious on a terrace in beautiful surroundings? This is pure delight.

From this time in Tirol, I still remember what an older golf player said to his wife, 'But dearest, if you always chip so nicely you will never really learn to putt.'

'I WOULD NEVER HAVE EXPECTED THE GAME TO BRING ME SO MUCH JOY.' – EVA B

It is twenty-five years now since I lost my heart to the wonderful landscape, the history and the traditions of England and Scotland during our summer holidays there.

At numerous golf clubs, I watched people who arrived directly after work, changed out of their working clothes and happily started playing a round of golf with their friends. I was fascinated – I also wanted to have a hobby like that. I did not know anything about golf rules – the only thing I knew was that in Switzerland golf was considered a sport for show-offs and rich people. I did not want to play there – I wanted to enjoy it in tranquillity and peace, as was the tradition on the island.

My husband and I drove to a golf club in England where I wanted to start playing at once. The man in the pro shop asked: 'What is your handicap?'

I was nonplussed because I did not know what he was talking about. But without this handicap, I was not allowed to play. I was disappointed, but at least I managed to play some 'pitch & putt' with my husband and sons and finally had a club in my hands.

Then, I buried my wish and twenty years passed.

When the golf course in Rheinfelden was built, I did not take any notice at first. But my sister and her husband from Austria started playing golf. Now all the talk was about golf and golf adventures, and I had nothing to contribute.

My Nordic walking tour took me along the golf course almost every day. One day, I gathered all my courage and asked at the pro shop how I could start playing golf. With a friend, I enrolled for a beginners' course in 2013. I was very pleased that Andrew Cullen from Scotland was the pro in Rheinfelden then. I have stayed with him till today. I admire his endless patience, his fine sense of humour and above all his sharp eye. After a couple of practice swings, he can always tell me what I do wrong and usually I understand it immediately.

I was not aware how much patience, practice and especially time I needed until my golf balls started flying more or less in the direction I wanted them to go in. Unfortunately, this does not always happen, even today.

I would never have expected the game to bring me so much joy. It has become a must-have on my holidays, and I have met many like-minded golfers. I like the peace, the concentration, the challenge and the possibility to forget everyday life. My holidays have an additional pleasure. Except during the winter holidays, my golf bag is always with me in the car or on the plane.

My husband does not play golf, but he supports me in my game. We go on holiday to Scotland every year, where I can choose from the most beautiful and quiet courses. I prefer old links courses to the modern golf courses in Europe – like the 'Cullen Links Course' on the Moray Firth that was designed by Old Tom Morris in 1875.

My life has got richer from these new experiences. Since retiring, my free time is filled with a sport that brings me many happy moments.

Health benefits

As I enter my fifty-sixth year on Planet Earth as Andrew Cullen, as fit, if not fitter than I've ever been, I am reminded of how big a role playing golf for the past fifty-three of those years has played in maintaining this healthy mind and body. Playing golf outside in the sunshine and fresh air, walking at a pace of 6-7km/h for several hours and constantly challenging the brain to perform complex physical playing tasks, makes golf one of the healthiest games on the planet – an antidote to the modern trend towards sedentary lifestyles and high stress working environments.

So, if you were contemplating taking up golf but thought you'd wait till you retire, think again. I recommend that you check out www.golfandhealth.org for a comprehensive look at golf's most important physical and mental health benefits, but here's a brief overview of how golf will not only help you get healthily to retirement, but also prolong your time and enjoyment in retirement![5]

Heart health

Any light physical activity which raises the heart rate is known as a preventative tool against cardiovascular disease, which is responsible for over 30% of worldwide deaths annually.[6] I encourage everybody I teach to walk the golf course as opposed to hiring a buggy. It's not only part and parcel of the sport but also contributes to a healthy heart.

Mental health

The pleasure of walking in fresh air, being in a natural environment, socialising, and challenging the brain in play situations, means golf releases endorphins – the natural mood-enhancing chemicals in your brain, which aid relaxation and happiness. In combination with physical activity, this can have a positive effect on reducing stress, depression and anxiety and can help individuals improve their confidence and self-esteem.[7]

Weight loss

The generally accepted daily requirement for weight loss of 10,000 steps is easily surpassed when walking 18 holes of golf, burning up to 2,000 calories.[8]

Improved sleep

Exercise and fresh air are a powerful combination for improved sleep. Walking the course and engaging the brain will give you a good physical and mental workout. Performed regularly, golf can help you go to sleep faster, remain in deep sleep longer, and assist muscle rest and repair.

Low injury

No physical activity comes with zero risk of injury, but golf is certainly a low-risk, low-impact sport. Golfing injuries include elbow, knee joint and lower back pain. However, warming up properly, having good technique and wearing and using good equipment should protect you from the majority of golfing injuries.

Live longer

In their study, 'Golf: a game of life and death – reduced mortality in Swedish golf players', the Karolinska Institute, Sweden, found that golfers have a 40% lower death rate, which corresponds to a five-year increase in life expectancy.[9]

> 'We know that the moderate physical activity that golf provides increases life expectancy, has mental health benefits, and can help prevent and treat more than 40 major chronic diseases such as heart attacks, stroke, diabetes, breast and colon cancer. Evidence suggests golfers live longer than non-golfers, enjoying improvements in cholesterol levels, body composition, wellness, self-esteem and self-worth. Given that the sport can be played by the very young to the very old, this demonstrates a wide variety of health benefits for people of all ages.'[10]
>
> —**Dr Andrew Murray,** Lead Researcher, Golf and Health Project, Physical Activity for Health, Research Centre at the University of Edinburgh

Most golfers I know will tell you that they wish they had taken up the game at a much younger age and that they had found a good professional instructor to help them build solid swing technique from day one. I hope I can start to dispel some of the common barriers to taking up golf, extol the many merits of this game, guide you step by step to a great golf game, and at the very least encourage you to read further and give it a go on your local driving range, pitch and putt, backyard or wherever! Now, let's move on in your journey to play the greatest game on the planet (my totally biased opinion... and I'm proud of it!).

Golden nuggets

- Learn to play golf for the joy it can bring you. The challenge, the health benefits, the social interaction, the stress release, the environment, the club atmosphere, the competition: there is a smorgasbord of delights that await you in a sport you can play for life.

- I hope that you will come back to this page in a few months' or years' time and say, 'This chapter was my golden nugget. This is why I started playing golf.' I would be honoured!

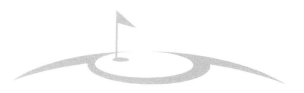

CHAPTER 2

What Do I Need To Learn?

When I first moved to Switzerland in 2003, one of my tasks as the head pro at Golf Club Limpachtal was to create and write up the content for a series of courses we were offering our students – full swing technique, putting, bunker play, short game and one of my favourites, 'trouble shots'. In this latter course, we explained, demonstrated and coached our students on how to play from sloping lies, rough grass, fairway bunkers and other awkward lies that one can experience during a round of golf. At the time, there were three pros delivering the courses, so it was important to have a written content reference to keep our coaching consistent. The evening before one of the Saturday 'trouble shots' courses, Boris, a Slovenian pro with pretty good English, said to me, 'Andrew, I have trouble shots course tomorrow and I don't know what to do'. I looked at him, puzzled, and replied, 'But Boris, it's all written down in the courses file. Just follow that.' His perplexed look remained, and he said, 'Yes, I know, but do you see who's on the list for this course? For these peoples, every shot is trouble shot!'

In case you are unacquainted with how golf is played, here's a quick overview:

- A golf course usually consists of 9 or 18 holes.

- Each hole has a start point (the tee) and a finish point (the hole).

- The aim is to play the ball from the tee into the hole in as few shots as possible.

- Each hole is a different length usually ranging from 100 m or more to over 500 m.

- Most holes are made up of the teeing ground (tee), fairway (short-cut grass) and rough (longer grass), and they may also have bushes, trees and hazards: bunkers (large holes in the ground filled with sand) and water hazards (eg rivers, streams, lakes, drainage channels). The hole is cut into a green: an area with very short-cut grass and often with undulations.

- Every golf course is different. Almost every country in the world has golf courses. (Awesome!)

Sounds pretty simple: hit it, find it, hit it again and do that as few times as possible on every hole. But this game is a great challenge and multi-faceted. That's why it's so much fun and pushes the mind and body to perform extraordinary tasks. Take, for example, the physics of hitting a ball with a golf club with a full swing and the ball landing on the green.

It's pretty mind-boggling. Wield the golf club, weighing 500 g, around your head and then swing the club at the ball with as much speed as you can generate. The 8 cm clubhead must make contact at or under the equator of a 4.3 cm diameter ball for it to fly. On making good contact, the ball ascends with backspin and sidespin characteristics (affecting its trajectory and direction), dependent on the angle (loft) of the clubface and the direction in which you swung the clubhead at the ball. The ball is subject to outside forces of wind strength and direction, air temperature, humidity and density, which all affect its flight characteristics. The ball's reaction on landing – bounce and roll – is dependent on the backspin the ball has left, the softness or hardness of the green on which it has landed, the length of the grass, the slope direction and the moisture of the grass surface. Oh, and there may also be an elevation difference between you and the flag to factor in.

To perform these feats of physics, you need a good, repeatable technique and rhythm, you need to develop your eye-to-ball coordination, and you need to trust your amazing brain and body. You cannot consciously compute all the physics of the exercise as described. Every second of every minute of every day, your brain is making thousands of computations to perform every conscious or subconscious movement that you make, such as determining which muscles to engage to stop you from falling over. You didn't have to read a book on how to walk when you were a baby; instead, you fell over a lot, and that helped your brain and body to work it out. They will also start to work out how to make contact with the little ball that's lying on the ground waiting for you. The point of coaching golf technique is assisting your brain and body to bring you to proficiency quickly and build a powerful, healthy, rhythmic and repeatable swing. It's like getting a baby to dance!

Below is my list of what you need to learn to get started. Most of the items are not in any particular order, but getting proficient at striking the ball with your club swing will probably take the longest time so I've made it the top item of the list:

- Full swing: How to swing a club powerfully, efficiently and without injury, connect with the ball, and send it in the desired direction

- Playing with different clubs to vary distance and trajectory

- Rhythm: Sequencing the swing movement and giving your brain an easy task

- Practising effectively: Maximise improvement in your technique, tempo and preparation for playing on the golf course

- Approach: Reduced swing from under 100 m to the green

- Bunker: Easy-out sand play from fairway and greenside bunkers

- Putting essentials: Direction control, distance control and reading the green

- Etiquette and rules: The bare minimum knowledge needed to enjoy your game

- Concentration and positive thinking: Training your brain to perform consistently at your best

- Fit to swing: Mobility exercises to improve your swing and prevent injury

There have been countless books written about each of the above topics, and I encourage you to read and learn further from qualified professionals. This book, and the accompanying online learning platform, are your one-stop shop to get quickly and enjoyably into the game, and the following chapters will introduce you to the above elements.

How long is it going to take?

It's a question I'm often asked, and fear of a big-time commitment can be a reason or excuse for not taking up golf. My answer: it's different for everyone. I know that's not the answer you wanted to hear, but it's the truth – and you know now that I only tell the truth! There are many factors to consider:

- **How is your mobility?** I've worked with young athletes and octogenarians with double hip replacements. Everyone can play; but, as in most sports, good joint mobility enhances the ability to make a powerful, repetitive, healthy movement, which can speed up your progress in golf. The good news: everyone can increase their mobility through exercise.

- **How much time do you have to practise?** If time is an issue, there are exercises you can do at home to build a good swing movement (see the 'HIIT training for golf' sections in relevant chapters). However, there is no substitute for swinging at and connecting with the ball to build your coordination.

- **Have you played other ball sports?** Particularly, if you have played or still play tennis or baseball, you're off to a great start. They require similar movements, and you'll already know how to swing at a ball.

- **Do you play any other sports** or otherwise keep fit to develop your body awareness? I'm a big fan of Pilates and yoga for helping your golf swing and calming your mind. They both deal with core strength, which is essential for body stability and helping protect the back, as well as balance and breathing, also important elements in the golf swing.

- **How's your concentration?** If you can't maintain focus for long, I'd recommend short but frequent practice sessions. If you have a good concentration span, you can put in longer, more effective practice sessions.

- **How is the rest of your life?** What demands do family, work hours, other commitments, sleep, nutrition, other hobbies or pastimes, and stress place on you?

So, if you're a former tennis player with good mobility, have plenty of time and energy to practise, have a good concentration span, and have no work or social commitments or stresses, then, firstly, you're not normal, and, secondly, you could probably play golf proficiently in a week! At the other extreme, if you're awaiting two hip replacements, have no time or energy to practise, have never played ball sports before, are not fit, have the attention span of a goldfish and have such a stressful life that you never sleep, then I'll have to re-invent the 'no hope category' I'd dismissed in Chapter 1. Most of you will lie some-where in between these examples and we can go ahead with learning to play golf. I reckon most of you reading this will need anywhere between a few weeks and a few months to gain proficiency and enjoy-ment, given effective practice sessions.

In the initial learning phase, you must ensure that you:

- Have a clear concept and picture of what you are trying to do

- Are developing your feel for good positions and movement through practising effectively

- Feel a curiosity to learn that outweighs your frustration

- Take great joy in the good, if somewhat sporadic, initial results

Personally, if I'm learning something new, I'm not satisfied with the 'Just do it this way because it works' teaching approach. I need logic and reasoning. That is what I deliver, and aim to always improve on, in my daily work as a coach. I'm convinced that the pupil who has clarity and intention in their learning has more potential than the pupil who hopes to stumble across the magic ingredient.

The tools of the trade

The equipment and materials used to play golf have changed dramatically since its inception in fifteenth-century Scotland. The 'sticks' have changed from wooden-shafted and -headed clubs with leather handles to high-tech steel- or carbon-shafted clubs with multi-material heads (commonly steel, carbon, titanium and tungsten) and rubber grips; balls made of leather stuffed with feathers have given way to multi-layered polymer balls. Although golf's ruling bodies put performance restrictions on golfing equipment, the ingenuity of golf's leading manufacturers in extending how far and straight the ball will go knows no bounds. At the top professional level, this is a continuing problem for the integrity of the sport; for the other 60 million of us who play golf, this is awesome! Make the game easier to play, get results faster and increase the enjoyment? Hell yeah!

However, I should emphasise the word 'easier'. It's a relative term. Golf is easier to play now than it was when I first started in the late 1960s, let alone back in the fifteenth century, but 'easy golf'? Classic oxymoron. That's all part of the challenge and fascination. The player wielding the stick, whatever it's made of, still has to do it with skill and dexterity. Good equipment will help you, but it doesn't swing itself.

As with many sports, the beginner is faced with a bewildering array of equipment to choose from. Golf may be one of the most complex sports in this context because it requires more than one 'stick'. Most golf sets consist of irons, woods, hybrids, wedges and a putter – pretty confusing, so I'll explain why we need different clubs and then recommend what you'll need to get started.

Take a look at Figure 1. Hitting the ball different distances with the same swing is a geometry exercise – a long-shafted club will create more radius and therefore more speed than a short-shafted club. By altering the loft (or angle of the clubface) in addition to the length, the distance a proficient golfer can hit with each club varies by around 10 m (eg 7 iron = 120 m; 8 iron = 110 m; 9 iron = 100 m).

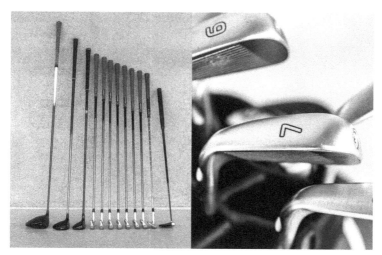

Figure 1
7 Iron and golf set

A typical set will contain:

- Irons 5, 6, 7, 8, 9, PW (pitching wedge) and SW (sand wedge): The PW and SW are mostly used for short approach (see Chapter 6) and bunker shots (see Chapter 7).

- Hybrids and fairway woods: Although irons 2, 3 and 4 are generally still available, they are difficult to get airborne for the beginner. The shape of the clubhead changes in the longer clubs to allow weight distribution and centre of gravity positioning to assist in getting the ball high from low-lofted clubheads. So, to play longer distances from the fairway we have hybrids and fairway woods.

- Driver: The driver is the longest and least-lofted club in the bag and is only used from the teeing ground with the ball teed up.

- Putter: The putter is used on the green to roll the ball towards and into the hole.

The bare minimum: 7 iron, SW, putter

If you're not sure whether golf is for you yet, and you don't want to invest too much money on equipment, but you need something to use at the driving range, I recommend getting a 7 iron, SW and putter. The 7 iron will go far enough when struck well to give you the 'Wow!' factor but its length is manageable enough to quickly develop your eye-to-ball coordination. The SW is adaptable for approach and bunker play, and you need a putter to play on the greens.

Recommended set: driver, fairway woods 5 and 7, hybrid 4, irons 5–9, PW, SW and putter

If I've already convinced you to 'golf yourself to life', get yourself a good quality set of new or used clubs. At the end of this book, I have listed my 'Recommended Golf Equipment Suppliers'. Having worked for many years with these manufacturers and sites, I know and trust them. Alternatively, you can go to a PGA pro based at a golf club or a good golf store for advice on what equipment would best suit your needs.

Ready for action? Then let's crack on into the following chapters with enthusiasm and curiosity!

Golden nuggets

☞ Your 'to do' list in learning to play golf – all the subjects covered in this book and the supporting online course:

- Full swing

- Playing with different clubs

- Rhythm

- Practising effectively

- Approach

- Bunker

- Putting

- Etiquette and rules

- Concentration and positive thinking

- Golf-fit

☞ In the initial learning phase:

- You should have a clear concept and picture of what you are trying to do

- Try to develop your feel for good positions and movement through effective practice

- Your curiosity to learn should outweigh your frustration

- Take great joy in the good, if somewhat sporadic, initial results

☞ Get equipped: start with a minimum of a 7 iron, SW and putter

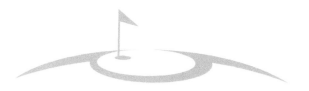

CHAPTER 3

Full Swing

'OK, I'm ready to learn – let's start.'

By the age of 15, I was golf mad. I had followed the careers and had the books of the two greats of that era (the 1970s), Jack Nicklaus and Tom Watson. I sat mesmerised in front of the TV in 1977 as these two giants battled it out in one of the great Open Championships of all time at Turnberry, later to be known as 'the duel in the sun'. But in 1980, there was a new kid on the block – an Australian. Tall, handsome and athletic with snowy, long blond hair. An icon: Greg Norman. The British Open Championship – often referred to simply as 'The Open' – the oldest of the four major golfing Championships (the others are the US Open, USPGA and the Masters) and the only one to be held in the British Isles, was at Muirfield near Edinburgh that year, and my dad had tickets. It was a dream for me, seeing all the greats of the time on the driving range, like Trevino, Crenshaw, Watson and Nicklaus, and watching the balls, one after another, sailing off into the sky from seemingly effortless swings. And then it was onto the golf course to follow the great champions as they battled against the challenging east-coast golfing links.

It was on the 6th tee, a 458-yard par 4, that I first experienced the sight and sound of the most powerful swing of that golfing era from the legend in the making, Greg Norman. At that time, the players were still using wooden-headed clubs to tee off. The sound from the Persimmon was best described as a soft cracking thump as wood contacted ball. First to tee off in the three-player group was young Englishman Paul Way. He was a fine player and played a beautifully drawing (right-to-left spin) drive, high over the bank, 100 yards in front of the tee and into the middle of the fairway. The closest spectators, a golf-savvy lot, offered a gentle applause and encouragement. Next up, and eventual winner of The Open that year, the great Tom Watson. Again, a lovely crack-thump from the Persimmon, and then extended applause and cries of 'Gawn, Tom!' The thrifty golfing Scots knew where to put their money that week. And then stepped up 'the Great White Shark', as he later became known due to his white locks and ferocious shots. There is an aura about great people which is often indescribable. It's something to do with their posture, their movement, their mannerisms, their chosen words, and the way their clothes look as if they were all tailor-made for them. Norman had it. You could almost sense the grass bowing down in respect to the great man. He took up a poised, athletic position, gave the club a little waggle and made a slow deliberate backswing. The next sound was like a cowboy's whip being cracked against a simultaneously exploding skull! The crowd gasped rather than applauded at the hellish sound. Nobody saw where the ball had gone as it had whistled off with such speed and height that it was virtually un-trackable with the naked eye. This was new. Mr Norman was a game changer.

I was fortunate to obtain Greg Norman's first instructional videos when I started my apprenticeship in 1988. That was a huge influence for me. Of course, I wanted to be a great player, but those videos were the platform for my teaching career. Athletic posture, soft hands, body rotation, arm speed and coordination of movement – this was as logical a description for a golf swing as I'd ever heard, and powerful! This was the future.

Swinging/throwing motion

Let's dive in and build your golf swing. By 'full swing', I mean trying to create as much speed in the club as you can to propel the ball as far as possible in the desired direction. The golf swing for me consists of three tasks: Firstly, a throwing motion of the club; secondly, a connection with the ball; and thirdly, sending the ball in the desired direction. As I am sure you are aware, multitasking is rarely easy. The size of the golf ball, a mere 4.27 cm in diameter, makes combining the three tasks a great challenge, particularly since the ball will only fly when you contact it somewhere under its equator; that means you're aiming at a 2.135 cm target.

While task one is a throwing motion, you need to decide which side to throw from, left or right. In my experience, you'll progress quicker, have a more natural club throwing motion sequence and more potential to reach a higher standard of play when you come from your stronger side. I've taught many exceptions to this rule, particularly many ice hockey players who have developed great coordination from their 'weaker' side. But we want to make this as simple as possible, so let's stick to your strong side. If you're not sure which side is your stronger side, or are ambidextrous, just go out and throw a few balls from each side, decide which feels better and stick with it.

Now for a little club throwing theory. As I mentioned in Chapter 2, in my experience the student armed with a clear picture of what they're trying to do will progress quicker and be able to practise more effectively and independently than the student who has no prior knowledge or who is told what to do without any supporting 'why'. So, pay attention – this is one of the keys to your quick progress. When you throw a ball, stick, javelin or whatever, there is a distinct sequence of movement to pass energy that the body creates both on its own and how it reacts with the ground, to the object being thrown, to propel it as far as possible. For example, the baseball pitcher sequence is (see Figure 2):

1. Body turns side on to target

2. Body continues turning motion away from the target and weight transfers to the back foot

3. Arm set behind the body, followed by body movement towards the target

4. Weight increasing on the front foot, with more pressure into the ground under the front foot bringing a straightening of the front leg leading to rotation of the lower body

5. This is followed by rotation of the upper body, then by leverage and rotation of the arm before releasing the ball (or whatever) from the hand

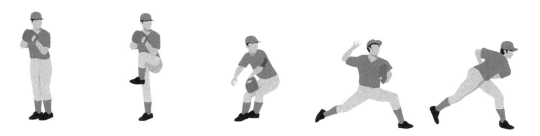

Figure 2 *Baseball pitcher throwing sequence*

It's amazing to watch professional baseball pitchers perform this sequence, throwing baseballs faster than 150 km/h.

When we introduce a club (for golf) or racquet to this throwing motion, we see the same sequence but with a distinct 'club' swinging direction (see Figures 3 and 4):

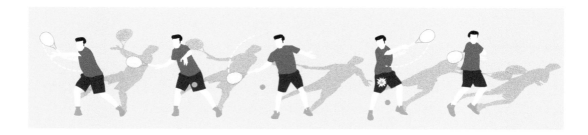

Figure 3 *Tennis player forehand sequence*

1. Hold the club or racquet upright (relative to the ground) on the turn away from the target

2. Flatten the club swing at the start of the downswing (which holds and sometimes increases the arm leverage and rotation)

3. Bring the club to a right angle relative to the upper torso, making the transfer of energy from the torso rotation to the club efficient (and putting less strain on the arm or arms)

4. Follow the shot through across the body

5. Continue the swinging motion around the body

In summary, an upright swing of the racquet behind the body, to a flatter and rounded motion to strike the ball and beyond. What I call an 'upright to flat to around' motion (see Figure 4).

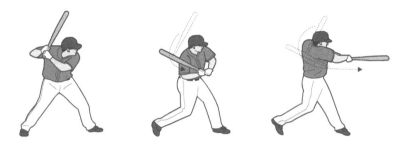

Figure 4 *Baseball batter swing sequence*

If you can incorporate this natural and efficient club/racquet 'throwing' direction into your golf swing development before we get into the details of the exercise, then you'll have great golf-playing potential.

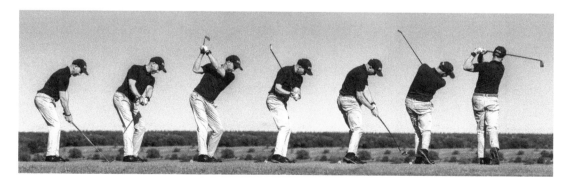

Figure 5 *Golfer swing sequence*

So, let's keep this concept and picture of how the club swings, transferring energy from the body and arms into speed in the club, and direct this motion at the ball that's lying on the ground waiting for you.

Practice tip: Upright to flat to around

Go whack some stuff with a stick, play fetch with the dog, hit some tennis balls or baseballs and develop your awareness of throwing or swinging a stick or club: Where is the club in relation to your body? What do you notice about your body movement, arm movement, tensions and sequencing? Don't get too technical, just be aware of how you naturally create speed in the club or stick.

Posture

This is massive. Get your posture right, and your body will rotate, react with the ground and stay stable without too much effort. Get it wrong, and you're in for a series of compensations, weaknesses and maybe injuries in what will be a contorted, inefficient throwing motion.

I mention the 'throw' of the club often as this is the feeling I want you to get. Obviously, you are going to do some damage if you actually throw the golf club, so keep hanging on to the club but maintain a light grip pressure. We'll talk more about the importance of this later in this chapter and in Chapter 10.

We need to direct this 'throw' of the club downwards towards the ball, so let's get into golfing posture. If you stand relaxed and upright, there are three natural positions you want to keep in your golf posture (see Figure 6):

1.   The relationship of your head to spine should be a straight line or in its natural 'S' form. If you naturally have a bit of a hunch or your head protrudes forward a bit, it's not ideal but maintain it in your golf posture.

2.   Your shoulders and upper body should be straight, or you should feel the distance between your shoulder blades. If your shoulders naturally sit forwards of your upper torso, again it's not ideal but maintain this in your golf posture.[*]

3.   A slight knee flex. It's important to note that we stand naturally neither with locked-out knees or very bent knees. This slight knee flex will also be maintained in the golf posture.

---

*   In my experience working with golf physiotherapists and osteopaths, one can improve these positions with massage and exercises. I recommend consulting such professionals if this is pertinent to you.

To get into golfing posture, you need to bend forward with the upper torso from the hip joint to direct the throwing motion of the club towards the ball. If you're wondering how much to bend, here's a great three-point check:

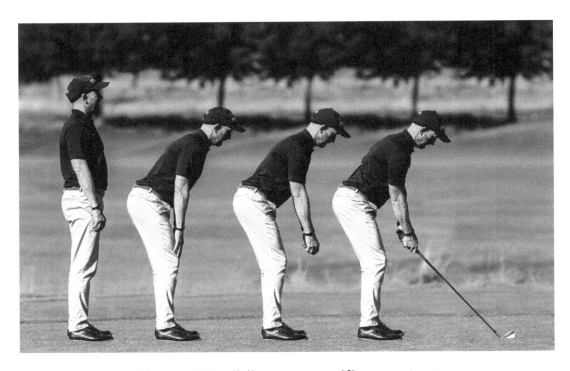

Figure 6 *Building your golfing posture*

1. Place your hands flat on the fronts of your thighs while standing in a relaxed upright position

2. Bend forwards from the hip joint, taking care not to adjust any of the three natural positions (head to spine, shoulders to upper torso, knee flex) until the tip of your longest finger touches the top of your kneecap

3. Let your hands hang under your shoulder joints

That's it: perfect golf posture – athletic and ready to rotate, stay stable and balanced, put pressure into the ground, and throw the club down towards the ball with a powerful, efficient, consistent and injury-free motion.[*]

In my experience, this check works for about 90% of people, across all body types and shapes and genders. Occasionally, someone with particularly long or short arms upsets the theory a fraction, but it doesn't take much adjustment to get in a great athletic position. Positive feedbacks to look for are a little tension in your gluteus maximus (your butt) and pressure in the ground under your shoelaces. If the tension is in your lower back, don't swing! It's not good for the lower back to tense the muscles and rotate, or to contract or extend the lower spine and rotate.

[*] I learned this from Mike Adams – a world-class golf biomechanics teacher: mikeadamsgolf.com

Adjust the knee flex or stand more upright till the tension is in your glutes and maybe also in your hamstrings (depending on your flexibility).

A lot of my 'first lessons' with experienced golfers are centred around getting their posture natural and orientated towards the ball. This has a massive positive effect on how the body, arms and club move and how the body can stabilise and balance. Check this position often in your mirror at home or on the driving range. I cannot emphasise enough the importance of posture in your golf swing development – that's why it is very deliberately number two on my full-swing list after 'how to swing a club'. Now, let's move on to how to grip the club.

Grip

Before we get into the grip, I want to apologise to all left-handers from this point onwards. To avoid confusion and unnecessary parentheses and lengthy explanations, all descriptions will be for the right-handed golfer. All lefties, please work with the mirrored position. According to golf industry experts, around 5-7% of golfers in the North American market are left-handed,[11] but this figure has many regional differences – for example, from my experience of working in Switzerland and Canada, there are proportionately more left-handed players than the expected 5-7% due to the influence of ice hockey. And, unusually, in the highlands of Scotland there are also more 'lefties' due to the influence of Shinty – a brutal hockey-based sport played with a double-sided hitting surface. But most golfers are right-handed; therefore, for ease of writing I shall proceed with right-handed explanations.

Many golf instruction books will put grip as number one on their list of swing factors. It is, after all, your only contact with the club. Many will also state that the hands must be in a very particular position. Well, I have seen a lot of pretty awful swings from 'textbook' grip positions, and some pretty amazing swings from non-textbook positions, and everything in between. What is important, as with posture, is that we keep the grip as natural as possible. So, let's build your grip.

Grab your 7 iron and build your posture as explained in the 'posture' section. Let your arms hang down as relaxed as possible. You'll notice that your hands turn in a little and they don't lie parallel to each other. How much they turn in varies from person to person. Now, build your grip (see Figure 7):

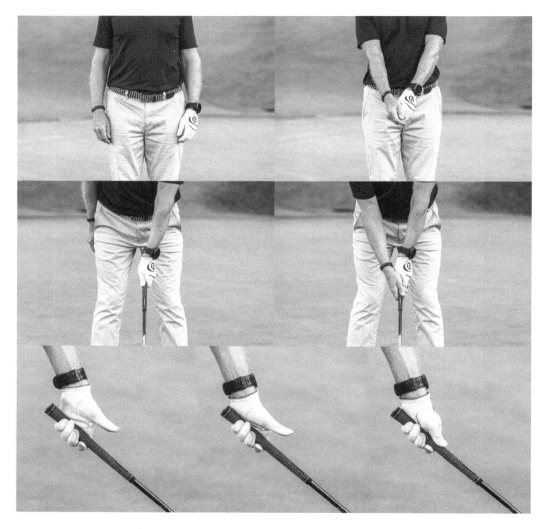

Figure 7 *Building your grip sequence*

1. Try to maintain your naturally turned-in position and place your left hand on the club, wrapping your fingers around the club and pointing your thumb down towards the clubhead. I'm going to talk more about this top-hand position in Chapter 10 as it's critical in the throwing motion, how the arms coordinate with your body movement, and the relationship to the clubhead position at impact with the ball.

2. Place your right hand on the club below, and as close to the left hand as possible. You'll notice it's a little more difficult to keep your turned-in position as the left thumb is in the way. For this reason, the palm of the right hand will sit more on the side of the club than the left hand, or parallel to the clubhead (refer again to Figure 7). You should feel a good fit between the heart line of your right hand and the side of your left thumb. The right-hand position affects the leverage of the right arm, which in turn has a big effect in generating club speed.

You have just built your basic grip position – what we call a baseball or 10-finger grip, as all fingers are on the club. I'd recommend you start with this grip for the first few times you swing. In Chapter 10, I'll introduce you to two adaptations of this grip, the interlock and overlap grip, which will help coordinate the left and right side. Even in those grips, however, the position of the hands will remain as I've explained above.

Alignment and ball position

The efficient, and desired, progression on the golf course is to play from the teeing ground to the fairway, the fairway to the green, and the green to the hole. Sounds easy, but I can feel the established golfers who are reading this already starting to grimace. To stand a chance of succeeding this way, you've got to aim; and the closer you get to the hole in this game, the more precise your aim has to be. Both how you align your body to your chosen target and where the ball is positioned in relation to your feet have an influence. My advice will be general here as how you move and how the club is moving will dictate how you align and where the ball position should be for you. You can adapt these positions later as necessary.

For alignment, imagine railway tracks (see Figure 8). Your ball-to-chosen-target (eg flagstick) alignment is one track, and you are standing on the other (ie parallel). Practise with sticks on the ground to get you into the habit of positioning yourself this way. The leading or lowest edge of the clubhead is aimed perpendicular to the railway track (ie straight at the target).

For ball position, the middle of the upper torso or sternum is your reference point. If you let your hands hang down from your golf pos-ture position and bring them together, they'll meet under the sternum. That's the low point of the hand swing and therefore the low point of the clubhead swing. And we want the clubhead to 'bottom out', ie

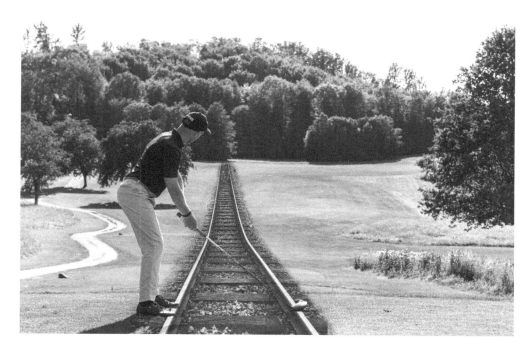

Figure 8 *Alignment*

reach the lowest point of its arc, at or just beyond the ball for a good strike. So, at the start the ball should be placed directly underneath where the sternum will be at strike. As we saw in the natural throwing motion, the body is moving forward on the downswing; therefore, in a good throwing motion of the club, the ball strike will occur anywhere between the middle of the feet and the heel of the front foot. For now, let's start by placing the ball underneath your sternum, or the mid-point between your feet, until you get some consistency of strike.

Before we test out your club swinging motion, golf posture and grip on the ball, let's get you warmed up to play.

Warm up before practice

First, a small word of warning. Repetitive strain injury (RSI) affects many activities, and golf is no different. We are trying to build a powerful, repeatable movement, after all. Golfers are particularly prone to elbow and forearm strain through repetition of movement and the tendency to hold the golf club too tightly. If you follow the above posture building correctly, you should avoid problems with the back, knees and shoulders, so getting warmed up before working on your swing technique is essential. It is more about injury prevention than just getting ready for movement.

I've seen some funky warm-up moves on driving ranges the world over in the past 50 years – proper potential trouser splitters. I wouldn't recommend them all but at least the golfer is getting their body ready to play. If you don't care a jot about what other people think – and I encourage this attitude – then, hell, throw some funky moves in there. The world needs entertainers. Rather than trying to follow a series of pictures, check out my 'Warm-up' video from the online video series accompanying this book (code on back page). These exercises are all designed to be done on the driving range or practice ground; none require lying on the ground or any potentially embarrassing manoeuvres, and they specifically involve warming up all the joints and muscle

groups involved in swinging the club. There are ma
tations and additions to these exercises, but I like to
simple and effective. We've come to the range to v
after all, not do a full aerobic session. In Chapter 8
home or gym exercises to help with your golf technic

Putting it all together

You're warmed up and ready for action – great! Let's start with your 7 iron or a short club – with the shorter clubs, it's a little easier to coordinate the movement and relation to the ball; if I gave you a tennis racquet that was 1 m long, you'd probably hit a few air shots! I'd also recommend hitting no more than 50 balls for the first few sessions; more balls would risk RSI. Start without the ball. Check your posture and grip positions and make some 'club throwing' motions, as described in the 'Swinging/throwing motion' section, while trying to make contact with the ground or driving range tee. If you're confident, pop a ball on the tee and see if you can make contact, concentrating on what you're doing to generate speed in the club. We never want to lose your natural ability to create speed in the club. Even if you miss the ball often at the start, stick to the priorities: 'throw the club'; get great posture to throw the club at the ball; and find your natural grip – this will help with speed and direction control.

Once you're done, I'd recommend repeating the forearm exercises from the warm-up to prevent elbow inflammation and muscle strains.

If you are like most beginners, you may have hit a handful of balls that have flown forwards somewhere, missed a few and 'topped' (hit balls but didn't make them fly) a lot. Maybe you even whacked the clubhead into the ground a few times. You're frustrated by the rubbish shots, but the ones that flew were fun. I can safely say, you're normal. So, why do some shots feel great and fly forwards and others just roll along the ground? Figure 9 shows what must happen to get the ball airborne.

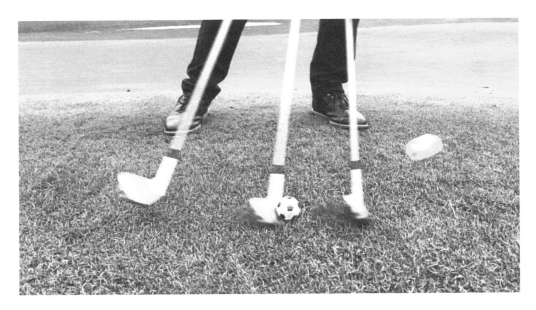

Figure 9 *Ball striking sequence*

If we 'throw' the club at the ball with speed, and the leading edge of the clubhead strikes the ball under its equator, the loft or angle of the clubface will launch the ball upwards and forwards with backspin, and bingo! Or, as Erika shared with us in Chapter 1, 'Wow! Shit! What a shot!' Brilliant.

'So, how do I do that all the time?' Well, I'd love to give you a simple answer. There are hundreds of theories, thousands of books and probably thousands of YouTube videos which endeavour to answer the beginners' ultimate question after yet another topped shot, 'What did I do wrong there?' And many teachers or well-meaning friends will offer tentative answers like, 'Just keep your head down', or 'Look at the ball', or 'Move the ball position', most of which are 'ball orientated' and not 'throw orientated'. The more you try to get the ball up in the air, the worse and more restricted the throwing motion becomes. Instead, let's breathe for a minute and get curious.

- The deliberate posture position we built will give you balance and stability as you swing the club around you. This stability, or distance control from the ball, will increase your likelihood of making contact with the ball.

- The club throwing motion of upright backswing, flattening on the downswing and moving around yourself to the finish will increase your chances of making contact with the ball.

- The grip position and light grip pressure, in combination with this 'throwing motion', will make you more likely to make contact with the ball.

- Keeping your eyes fixed on the ball during the throwing motion will also make you more likely to connect with the ball. *Very importantly*, keep watching the ball as it flies (hopefully) forwards; looking at the ground or where the ball was will restrict the throwing motion.

You'll notice I gave you no guarantees or quick fixes here – because there are none. This is a complicated movement, and we all move differently. Striking the ball consistently comes with executing the above and building your coordination to the ball through practice. The body, even in good players' swings, will move a few centimetres up, down and sideways relative to the ball position. We already know that we have only 2.135 cm of ball to aim at but staying absolutely still relative to the ball – ie not moving more than 2.135 cm away from the ball during the swing – while making this throwing motion is not only undesirable (because you won't make a good throwing motion) but physically impossible! So, we have to practise to allow our brain to interpret what we intend with our actions.

My answer to the question, 'What did I do wrong there?' would be, 'Well, let's talk about what you did right there. Were any of the three fundamentals (club throw, posture, grip) missing?' If the answer is 'No', then great! Keep practising and building your coordination to the ball. Your percentage of good shots will steadily increase as your brain and body work out the finer details – ie let the baby learn to walk through success and failure.

Try not to get too frustrated. There are many variables in the throwing motion which can influence how you strike the ball, and we will talk more about them in Chapter 10. For now, stick to the fundamentals and keep checking them. When you're having fun playing off a low handicap in a few years' time, you will thank me for this chapter.

Practise before moving on!

Rhythm

Now you've been to the driving range a few times with varying degrees of success (which is normal) and you're wondering what the next step is. Let's get some rhythm. Look back at the ball throwing sequence at the start of this chapter (Figure 2) and recall that there is a distinct sequence of movement to ball throwing, tennis, baseball and golf. The keys to this sequence in the forward motion are applying pressure in the ground under the front foot and 'releasing' the ball or club with the arm swing – a combination of arm rotation and elbow and wrist leverage. This requires stability and tension in the body (to move forwards and push in the ground) and, contrarily, a relaxation of the muscles in the hands, arms and shoulders (to achieve the release of the club). In the ball throw, for example, if we kept the fingers tight on the ball, the ball would not be thrown at all! Rhythm guides this sequencing, and I'll give you a few tips to get this sequencing as simply and naturally as possible.

Firstly, the body needs some tension to stabilise and create ground force. (By ground force, I mean your contact with and pressure into the ground. If you tried to play golf in sneakers on the ice, you'd quickly find out it's impossible – that's zero-ground force.) In creating your posture position, I mentioned getting some tension in your glutes as positive feedback. Keep these muscles engaged from start to finish in the swing. It not only provides for a powerful swing motion but will also help protect your back. If your glutes switch off, you're in for instability and poor ground forces. Also try lightly tensing the other core muscles – stomach (abs) and thighs (quads).

Secondly, the hands, arms and shoulders need to be relaxed to release the club properly. Release is the rotation of the arms (think tennis forehand) combined with the leverage of the trail arm (think hammer motion), which bends at the elbow and wrist on the backswing, creating leverage through the strike of the ball. This will happen naturally and subconsciously if the focus is on 'throwing' the club.

Ok, that was a slightly lengthy explanation for 'tighten your butt and relax your hands'. The rhythm (or sequencing) will come from keeping your grip pressure light and constant throughout the swing. If you find it hard to focus on your grip pressure during the swing, here are a couple of other rhythm helpers:

Breathe

It's amazing how many golfers hold their breath from start to finish during the golf swing. It's just as well we have relaxed walks in a beautiful environment between shots in this sport; otherwise, golf course fatalities would rise. Holding your breath is not good for the swing or your health, so keep breathing. Here are three methods to try:

1. Breathe in on the backswing and out on the downswing. Breathing out relaxes the muscles and will therefore help with the release of the club through your strike.

2. Breathe out during the entire swing. This obviously requires a good inhale before you start the backswing.

3. Keep your mouth slightly open and relax your face muscles to allow the breath to flow by itself without conscious effort.

Centre

If you are not getting anywhere with the above breathing suggestions, try centring. If you are familiar with yoga or Pilates, you'll know about centring. Your body centre is a point a few centimetres behind and below your navel. Focussing on and breathing into this point can improve your balance and also help clear your mind of busy thoughts or worries about getting the ball airborne. Your relaxed mind and body will create positivity and rhythm. It's a little more intangible than focussing on breathing but potentially much more powerful.

I've heard of other methods which can work to get good rhythm (eg humming, singing a song or starting the backswing slow), but you must work with your natural rhythm. It's much easier to repeat what comes naturally. If you speak fast, work fast and walk fast, you'll have a fast golf swing. That's fine, as long as the sequencing is correct, and you'll get that through constant light grip pressure or conscious breathing or centring. Experiment, see what gets the best results and stick with it!

Practise before moving on!

Concepts

I've kept the full swing technique general so far: throw, club swing direction, posture, grip and sequencing through finding your rhythm. I could happily leave it there and your ball-hitting consistency would naturally increase. But you could also develop some bad habits from experimentation or poor advice, so I want to give you some reference points. Feedback is critical in learning anything: Am I doing the right movement? Am I studying the right things? Am I pronouncing these French words correctly? (I'm constantly receiving feedback on the latter by my French partner, Gila, who sighs in dismay every time I utter a French expression with Scottish guttural 'cchhh' overtones.) Again, rather than filling your head with words or pictures, I encourage you to check out my videos relating to Chapter 3 in the video series accompanying this book. I also encourage you to download a sports video analysis app on your phone and film yourself to get positive feedback and identify weaknesses based on the concepts from my video series. The video series will give you a more detailed look at the main themes for developing a controlled throw of the club at the ball in the most efficient, powerful and injury-free way.

Get practising, get feedback, analyse what you have to improve and practise again – this is the learning cycle you must get into. You need to get curious to get good. I learned this too late in my career. I'd play a horrible round of golf, get upset with myself, huff and puff for hours (sometimes days), and when the frustration of not playing golf returned, I'd go and practise again. This is not the way to go. Don't get angry with yourself; this game is a big challenge. Play, analyse, plan what you need to improve, and then go and work on improving it.

You may have heard of the '10,000 hours practice to excellence', which sounds daunting.[12] The good news is that this is for 'mastery' of a skill; some amount of 'proficiency' is all we need to get great enjoyment from golf. I encourage you to read Josh Kaufman's book, *The First 20 Hours – How to learn anything fast* and view his TED talk of the same name. He breaks proficient skill acquisition into four stages:[13]

1. De-construct the skill – what we are doing in each chapter of this book.

2. Learn enough to self-correct – Use the information from this book in coordination with the online video series and videos of your own swing.

3. Remove practice barriers – ie distractions, like phone messaging or chatting with other people.

4. Practise for at least 20 hours – that's the equivalent of 45 minutes a day for one month.

'Deliberate practice' is the modern mantra. Whatever time you have in which to practise, give it your full attention, work at things that you or your coach have identified to increase your potential, and get feedback during practice to aid improvement. And have fun doing it! Positivity and fun enhance the learning process.

Practice suggestions

• Throw some sticks or golf clubs – **safely!** Be aware of, but don't try and influence, how the body is moving and the sequencing of the movement.

• Swing a golf club (without a ball) upright to flat to around. Upswing, upright; downswing, flat; around the body to finish.

- Swing a golf club (without a ball) upright to flat to around, aiming at a specific point or line on the ground. Aim to get the clubhead bottoming out at a consistent point.

- Introduce the ball to the point or line and have some fun!

- Keep checking your posture in a mirror.

- Keep checking your grip.

- Focus on keeping your grip pressure light and constant. Experiment with breathing and centring.

Golf HIIT – 10-15 minutes

HIIT in exercise training stands for 'high intensity interval training'. It is usually 10–15 minutes of intensive work and is for those who don't have the time or inclination to spend hours in the gym or at classes but are conscientious enough to do some regular exercise for the benefit that it brings. Many of my students have busy jobs or run their own businesses and have little time for golf practice – especially if they have young families – but they love their golf and want to get better. I recommend short practices that they can do at home, or in the back garden or garage, with and without a club and usually in front of a mirror, to help ingrain good positions or movement or feelings. It helps to build and strengthen the neural highways from brain to body part, which we want to use in each swing to access repeatability without conscious effort. It's often called 'muscle memory', but really, it's sending a consistent chemical and electrical message from the brain to the relevant muscle group(s). The more we use the same neural link, the more dominant it becomes through the build-up of myelin, which speeds up the chemical and electrical transmission.[14] I recommend reading Daniel Coyle's *The Talent Code* if you want to study how this works across sport, music and arts. If you fit into this group of time-starved professionals, or you just want to get better quick, then the golf HIIT in this book is for you!

Full swing HIIT[*]

- **10 × posture:** Re-read the 'Posture' section from this chapter. Build your posture ten times from a standing position in front of the mirror – front and side elevation.

- **10 × grip:** Re-read the 'Grip' section from this chapter. Build your grip ten times, taking your hands off the club after each attempt.

- **20 × upright to flat to around swing:** Study the tennis, baseball and golf swing sequence pictures from the beginning of this chapter. If you have the space, do this with a club. If you're indoors, do this with a short, rounded stick or similar that's about the same circumference as a golf club grip. Stand side-on to the mirror, take your posture, and grip and swing the stick as in the pictures from the 'Swinging/throwing motion' section of this chapter. Make sure

---

[*]   Some of the activities may not be high physical intensity but they are high focus intensity!

the downswing is flatter than the backswing. Ideally, the stick will swing at right angles to your spine on the downswing. Start with slow-motion swings and, as you see in the mirror that the movement of the stick is good, move up to full speed. The aim is to increase the 'whoosh' sound of the club or stick as it's swinging in front of you.

Golden nuggets

- Start and stay healthy, avoiding RSI. Warm up before each practice session to avoid injury and prepare the body to swing the club. Start with short sessions of up to 50 balls.

- Use the shorter clubs (eg 7, 8, 9 iron) that make it easier to coordinate your eye-to-ball distance.

- Focus at the start on 'throwing' the club properly: upright to flat to around.

- Check your posture, grip, alignment, and ball position often using feedback from a mirror or video.

- Find your rhythm: glutes and core lightly tensed; shoulders, arms and hands relaxed; experiment with grip pressure, breathing or centring.

- Get feedback during your session – from mirror work, video, body feels, ball flight – to progress quicker in the next session.

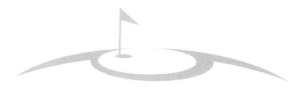

CHAPTER 4

Short Approach

'How do I get the ball on the green?'

There is a beautiful little town situated on a plateau in Valais in the Swiss Alps at approximately 5,000 feet above sea level called Crans Sur Sierre. One of the great highlights on the Championship golf course there is walking from the 6th green through a pine wood and past a few little holiday chalets to the 7th tee – and a breathtaking view of the Alps.

If you're ever in Switzerland, it's a 'must play' for its incredible vistas, technically challenging golf and the Swiss-speciality food served in the town. Never come to Switzerland without trying a good rösti! The golf course was witness, in the 1993 European Masters tournament, to one of the most creative and brilliantly executed golf shots that has ever been played. Not only that, but it was immediately followed by another. At the spot, among the pine trees to the right of the 18th fairway, where this great shot occurred now lies a plaque in honour of the feat. The player: the one and only, late, great Severiano (Seve) Ballesteros.

It was the fourth and final round of the tournament. Seve had just birdied the 13th, 14th, 15th, 16th and 17th holes in an incredible run of form and was one shot behind the leader, Barry Lane. He needed one more birdie to tie the lead and have a chance of winning the tournament. The 18th is a 350 m par 4 with a fairly severe left to right sloping fairway, running towards pine trees, out of bounds and a wall over which is the local outdoor swimming pool. Seve hit a terrible 3 wood shot straight right, which bounced down the slope and ended up 2 metres from the 2.5 m high swimming pool wall and surrounded by pine trees. Seve and his caddie Billy Foster – one of the best, wisest and most successful caddies there has ever been on the European Tour – found the ball and surveyed the situation. Billy is thinking, 'That's the tournament gone, but chip it out, wedge it on the green and you never know, still got a chance'. But Seve is down on his hands and knees looking up over the wall at a chink of daylight in the pine branches about 'the size of a dinner plate' – a route to the green. But, to compound the problem, he can only make half a backswing because of another pine tree behind his ball, and on his route to the green are more tall pine trees which he has to get over. It's an impossible shot. Billy sees what Seve is thinking and says, 'Seve, chip it out sideways, wedge it on the green and you can still hole the putt and win the tournament.' 'No, no, no, Billy, I see this shot, give me the pitching wedge.' After a few expletives, and a sarcastic reference to a famous British magician – 'You're not f-in Paul Daniels!' – Billy gives Seve the PW and returns, forlorn, to the fairway, expecting the worst: maybe he makes an 11, maybe 12. A caddie's income is a percentage fee from the prizemoney their player makes, so Billy is now spitting bullets. Seve looks up at the 'dinner plate', makes as much of a swing as he can at the ball, and a great puff of dust and pine needles is thrown up. Billy watches incredulously as the ball rockets over the wall, through the 'dinner plate' gap, sails over the pine trees bordering the fairway and lands 2 m short of the greenside bunker, a shot of some 120 m. Miraculous. Seve strolls up the fairway as if nothing special had happened, eyes up the chip shot over the bunker, takes the same PW and holes the chip for a birdie 3. Billy sinks to his knees and offers the worshipping bow.[15]

Imagination. Vision. Confidence. Implausible skill. Genius.

Unfortunately, it wasn't enough to win Seve the tournament. Barry Lane would win by one shot, but it was hallmark Seve: often wild off the tee, but a magician on approach play. It was a game plan that would win him ninety-one tournaments, including five major Championships. Beware the golfer with a great short game.

Part of the fascination and challenge of this game is its diversity. One minute, we are trying to send the ball as far as possible from the teeing ground to the fairway; the next, we have to play a 10 m shot over a water hazard to a hard and fast running green and get the ball stopping near the hole. In addition to good technique, we need feel, imagination and nerve, like the great Seve had in abundance. So, let's crack on with the next chapter in your golf development – short approach shots. Here's where the practice becomes real fun!

A short approach shot, for the purposes of this book, is anything less than a full swing shot played from outside the green and not in a bunker (see Figure 10). It is generally considered 100 m or less from the green. You'll read different definitions, particularly 'chipping' and 'pitching'. I'm not a lover of these two words as their definitions and technical content are often misinterpreted by both beginners and experienced players. For this reason, I'm not going to talk about them or give you the definitions, but please feel free to explore them.

The purpose of the short approach shot is to get the ball in the air and stop it on the green, hopefully near to or in the hole. The distance of this shot varies greatly; if you hit a full swing with a PW 70 metres, then a short approach shot with your PW is anything less than 70 m (ie it requires less than a full swing). What we are doing then is reducing the speed in the clubhead to send the ball less far than a full swing. The length of swing required for a set distance will also vary greatly from player to player depending on the speed they naturally generate – swing characteristics and rhythm – and the club they are using.

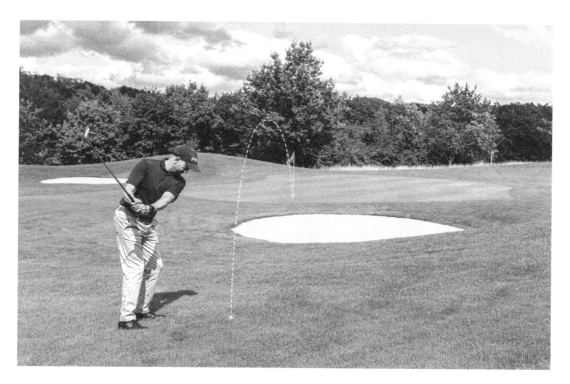

Figure 10 *A short approach shot*

Let's tackle this short approach shot systematically, looking at the following elements:

1. What needs to happen to get the ball in the air?

2. Swing characteristics

3. Set-up position

4.   Distance control

5.   Trajectory control

6.   Landing points and rolling out

7.   Longer approaches

What needs to happen to get the ball in the air?

I mentioned in Chapter 3 that to get the ball in the air, the leading edge of the club needs to make contact under the equator of the ball (see Figure 9). Ideally, we'll strike the ball in the sweet spot of the clubhead – the point on the clubface where the most efficient transfer of energy from the clubhead to the ball takes place – to get maximum control of the ball trajectory and spin and to get feedback or 'feel' from the ball strike. Therefore, the club needs to make contact with the ball at or just before the clubhead reaches its low point. If you take your golf posture position, letting your arms hang and with your hands together, without a club, and make a turning motion with your shoulders, you'll see that the low point of the hands' swing is always opposite your sternum; therefore, the low point of the club swing is also opposite your sternum. So, the sternum's position relative to the ball in the strike position is critical to get the ball airborne. We'll return to this relationship later in this chapter.

Swing characteristics

Here's the good news: we already have the swing characteristics from your full swing to apply to the short approach. We are trying to generate less speed, so we have less swing, but it's the same swing in a shorter form. To prevent the sternum from moving too far off the ball position, we keep the lower body stable on the backswing and the lower body will move with you on the down and through swing, but we don't need the power it brings in the full swing. The upper body controls the show here. The arms and hands stay passive and relaxed, and the upper body turns back and through, collecting the ball as the sternum moves forward with your turn through strike (see Figure 11). Keep it simple! If anyone advises you about using the wrists and arms in various ways, stick your fingers in your ears and give them the 'la la la' response. 'Turn and collect' is the feeling you're after. There are many adaptations we can make to this basic swing, but get this simple version installed early.

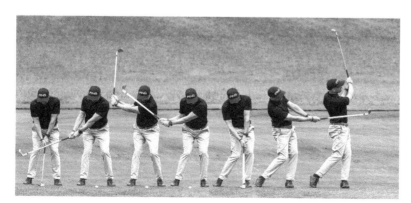

Figure 11

Short approach swing sequence

Set-up position

If you understand what has to happen to get the ball in the air, where the low point in the swing is, and how to make a simple repetitive swing with the upper-body turn, then the set-up logic is straightforward. Here's some more good news: the posture and grip are the same as in your full swing. Place the ball under or just in front of (target side) your sternum. The low point in the swing should come just in front of your sternum position at set-up if you keep your hands and arms passive and turn your upper body properly to make the swing. Again, a lot of advice will come your way (eg place the ball back in the stance, weight forward, use your wrists to get the ball up) – fingers in the ears, 'la la la'. Keep it simple, effective and repetitive. Adaptations, if necessary, can come later. All will be revealed.

Distance control

The easy way to control your distance is primarily with your swing length and secondly through constant rhythm. More distance requires more speed and therefore more swing. More swing means turning the upper body further and equally on both sides, backswing and fol-low-through. By keeping the rhythm the same, you only need to vary swing length. The easiest way to keep the rhythm constant is to keep your grip pressure constant. If you imagine a scale of 1–5 where 1 is as light as possible and 5 is as tight as possible, you want to be at 2 from start to finish. You can make adaptations to get more or less distance (eg change clubs, different ball positions relative to the sternum), but hold the phone! Let's get the basic shot correct and get consistency of ball strike and ball flight first. Then, you can start experimenting – and please do! Once you have the basics, it's time to get creative.

Trajectory control

You are going to need different shots to deal with the different situations you'll encounter around the greens, such as a high ball flight that needs to stop quickly to a flag position close to the edge of a bunker, or a low-ball flight that runs out a few metres to a flag at the back of a long sloping green (see Figure 12). You can deal with trajectory easily by keeping all the above basics the same and simply changing your club. Experiment here – try a 7 iron for a low flight, long running shot, a SW for a high flying, quickly stopping shot, or even have a go with the 6 iron, 5 iron or a hybrid.

Only rarely will you need to adapt something from this basic technique to get an especially high ball flight. (Tip: if you want the ball to fly higher than your SW shot, buy a lob wedge as it's more lofted than the SW.)

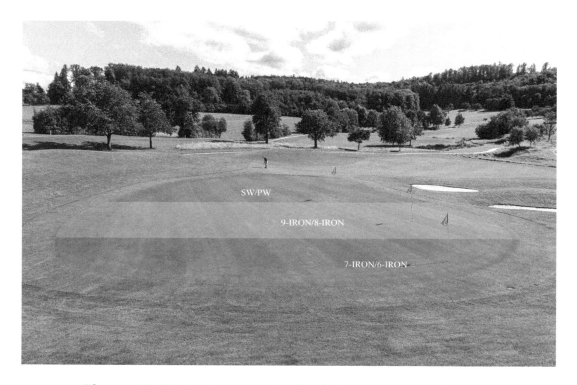

Figure 12 *Trajectory and roll of short approach shots*

Landing points and rolling out

Figure 12 is an extremely simplified version of the influence of club choice on trajectory and roll. Do not take for granted that, for example, the SW shot always flies 70% of the distance and rolls out 30%, or that the 7 iron flies 20% of the distance and rolls out 80%. It depends on the interplay of various factors, such as how fast the green is, the gradient of the green, how hard the ground is, the type of ball you are using, the wind strength and direction, rain or dew on the green, or whether you're playing from the fairway, semi-rough or rough. Oh, it's all part of the fascination and challenge of this incredibly important short approach shot. Experiment, experiment, experiment. There are no rights and wrongs here. It's about finding a way to get from where the ball is lying to as close to the hole as possible – or, indeed, in it. Short approach play, more than any other shot, requires a combination of good technique, good ball striking, good reading of all the conditions, good club choice and good visualisation. Did I say 'good'? I meant great!

As you'll discover in the chapter on putting, it comes down to reading the conditions of the situation and trusting your instinct. To get the ball close to the flag, how does the ball have to fly? How is it going to react with the ground? How is it going to roll out? Given all that, what club should I use and, most critically, where must the ball land? Now, imagine what the ball has to do, focus on the landing point, make a practice swing and feel the right swing with your chosen club, then trust your instinct and let it happen. Yep, you read it correctly: 'Trust your instinct and let it happen'. If I asked you to make a paper ball and throw it into your office bucket, would you study what you have to do with your hand and arm to get the paper ball in the bucket? Of course not. All the rehearsal is in practising your basics, reading the conditions and making good choices – club, trajectory, landing point. At some point, you have to give up control to the subconscious and let it happen.

Longer approaches

I hate lack of clarity, but it's difficult to define 'longer' in this context. A longer approach for a tour player could be 120 m, while for some players that's a good tee shot! It varies enormously from player to player. For the sake of clarity, I'll define it as a swing length at or longer than the 9 o'clock position on a clock face with the lead arm (left arm for right-handers), but short of a full swing (see Figure 13). Many players, even very good players, have trouble with this shot. If your arms and hands are overactive at the start of your full swing, you probably won't get any consistency with strike, direction and distance with this longer approach shot. So, once again, let's keep it simple! Try using this checklist:

1. Great posture (same as full swing)

2. Great grip

3. Grip pressure relaxed (see Chapter 3) – this is *essential*

4. Upper-body turn controls the show from start to finish.
    Feel yourself turn around your stable spine position

If you are turning your upper body well in both directions and maintaining a stable posture, the clubhead will again 'bottom out' opposite your sternum – at or just slightly target-side of the ball at strike. If your grip pressure is relaxed, your wrists will hinge automatically with the weight and momentum of the clubhead on the backswing and your

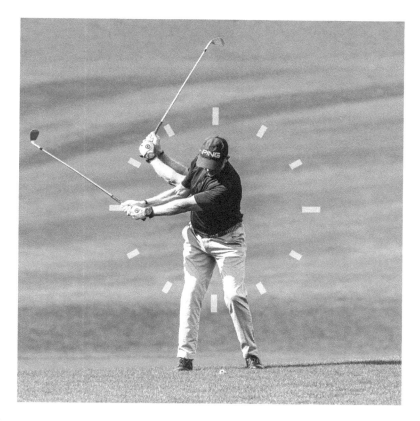

Figure 13 *9 o'clock and 10 o'clock longer approach swing*

sequencing will be good. This is not the only way to play this shot, but it's the simplest... and I did promise you simplicity! Enthusiasts may advise you to hinge your wrists early or hit down on the ball, but just remember your 'la la las'. Get your basics, and experiment later if necessary or if you're curious.

Once you get the ball consistently airborne with this longer approach shot, I recommend that you experiment with two swing lengths and different clubs: 9 o'clock and 10 o'clock with the lead arm – or waist height and chest height. Measure your average distance with a 9 o'clock swing with a PW, then do the same with a 10 o'clock swing; then, repeat with the SW so you end up with a little grid and four measurements. Once you get proficient and maybe have also a gap wedge and a lob wedge, you can add more measurements to the grid.

I see many mistakes from players of all levels with this shot. Many make their backswing the same length whatever the distance of the shot and stop turning their upper body on the downswing to slow the club down, placing their sternum in the wrong place at strike and making the club bottom out behind the ball. Others have a complicated wristy takeaway which loses control of the clubface and creates an arm swing that is independent of the upper-body turn. This can yield all sorts of results – few of them pretty. It's a tough shot; but keep it simple, be aware of your distances, and you'll realise quickly how important the approach shot is to your score on the golf course.

Practising short approach play

Technique: Start with short, simple swings with no specific target. Keep your upper body active and your lower body, hands and arms passive. The aims are consistency of ball strike, flight and developing feel.

Tempo: Ensure that your grip pressure remains constant from start to finish, whatever the length of swing.

Awareness: Play to different-length flag positions. Be aware of where the ball is landing and how far it is rolling out. Experiment with different clubs.

Landing point: Choose your landing point and focus on landing there as accurately as possible to get the ball stopping at the hole.

Experiment: Play from different lies and different distances, slopes, fairway grass, rough, etc, and with different clubs. Have some fun!

Approach HIIT – 10 minutes

- **10 × 9 o'clock to 3 o'clock swing:** With your club or indoor-work stick, take up your posture and grip face-on to the mirror. Swing the stick using only your upper-body rotation from 9 o'clock to 3 o'clock on an imaginary clock face (or parallel to the ground on both sides). Keep your lower half stable and your upper arms remaining at the sides of your body, as in the posture position. Stand out of your posture after each repetition and renew for the next swing.

- **10 × grip pressure #2:** Repeat the above exercise but focus on keeping the grip pressure constant at #2 (recall from this Chapter: grip pressure #1 is as loose as possible and #5 is as tight as possible). Take your hands off the club or stick after each repetition and renew for the next swing.

Golden nuggets

☞ The ball will fly if the leading edge of the club strikes underneath the equator of the ball

☞ Keep hands, arms and lower body passive, and upper-body turn active

☞ Keep posture and grip the same as for the full swing, with ball position under the sternum

☞ Control distance and trajectory through club choice and swing length

☞ Visualise your landing point and roll for precision play to the flag

☞ For longer approaches, stick to the checklist:

- Great posture

- Great grip

- Grip pressure relaxed

- Upper-body turn controls the show start to finish

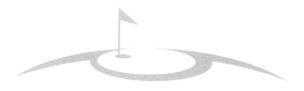

CHAPTER 5

Bunker Play

'Sand pits? Seriously? How do I get the ball out?'

In the late 1980s and early 1990s, the Bell's Scottish Open, one of the European Tour's big events, was played at Gleneagles. I love this place. The golf courses play in and around some breathtaking scenery. To play there in the evening with barely a soul on the golf course and an abundance of wildlife and colours and smells all around is golfing heaven – maybe even heaven full-stop. Mum, Dad and I used to travel up from Edinburgh to spend the day there and watch all the great players. That's when I first saw the legendary Severiano Ballesteros. As I mentioned in Chapter 3 with reference to Greg Norman, many great people have an indescribable aura about them, and Seve had it too. His posture, his handsome looks, his tanned skin and, as my mother pointed out on several occasions, his beautifully tailored trousers – everything about the man was remarkable even before you saw what he could do with a club and a ball.

It was the evening after the second round of a four-round tournament, and I was on the driving range to watch any players who felt that they needed to brush up their technique before the weekend. There were some Australian pros, including Brett Ogle and Peter Senior, passing the time and whacking a few balls. I was the only one there when the golfing magician, Seve, arrived and went straight to the bunker. 'What a treat!' I thought. 'I'm the only spectator here and I get to watch Seve live – not only the best golfer of this era but arguably the best bunker player of all time.' (Gary Player would probably argue with me on that one.) I sat and watched in awe as ball after ball popped effortlessly up high from the sand and landed softly on the green, nestling up to the hole as if it was a homecoming. The sound of the clubhead making contact with the sand was a soft, dull thud like I'd never heard before – like a wet sandbag being dropped from a height onto a tarmac road. Different distances, different flags, same result – the ball landed within a few centimetres of the hole, or, more than once, in the hole. It was a masterclass, with only one student: me.

So, what did I learn? The sound, as I later found out through my good friend and tour coach Jon Wallett, was the back edge of the sole of the club (or 'bounce') hitting the sand first. The effect is that the clubhead bounces back up off the sand from the impact, as opposed to digging into the sand. This creates less resistance from the sand and gives the speed of the clubhead to the ball, even though by bunker play the intention is to hit the sand before the ball. There was also a consistent and beautiful, unhurried tempo to the swing, coordinating the rotation of the upper body, arms, hands and club. These two features of Seve's bunker play, in addition to some basic principles, is what I'll endeavour to give you here so you too can be Master of the Sand!

Greenside bunker

There are greenside bunkers, next to or close to the green, and fairway bunkers. We'll deal with the latter in a later section of this chapter.

I'm going to keep this simple – surprise, surprise. As with other aspects of golf play, there are many adaptations one can make but my goal is to give you the confidence to get the ball out of the bunker with an element of distance control.

In the greenside bunker, we are trying to hit the sand behind the ball because direct contact with the ball, in most cases, will not generate enough height on the ball flight with a short swing to get the ball up and out of the bunker. And if there is any contact with the sand behind the ball with a short swing, the ball will stay in the bunker.

Set-up (see Figure 14)

We are going to keep the swing the same as the longer approach from Chapter 4 but set up to almost guarantee that you are going to whack the club into the ground behind the ball at speed. We try to avoid this at all costs with the long approach, but it will work perfectly for the bunker shot. The set-up adaptations are:

- Keep your ball position opposite the front foot.

- Put more weight, about 70%, on the front foot, which will make the swing steeper.

- Keep your hands positioned behind the clubhead.

- Clubhead addresses the ball 10 cm or so behind the ball so you can fix your eyes on a point in the sand behind the ball.

- Dig your feet into the sand a little. This gives you a little more stability, allows you to test the depth of the sand and brings you underneath the level of the ball.

These set-up positions help you to contact the sand first. Ideally, you are striking the sand first where your eyes are focussed – 5 cm behind the ball. The club bottoms out where the ball is resting and resurfaces 5 cm or so beyond the ball, so you are skimming the clubhead along the sand. Let me give you an analogy: imagine trying to splash a dollar-bill-sized area of sand out of the bunker – with the ball being placed in the middle of the dollar bill (see Figure 15).

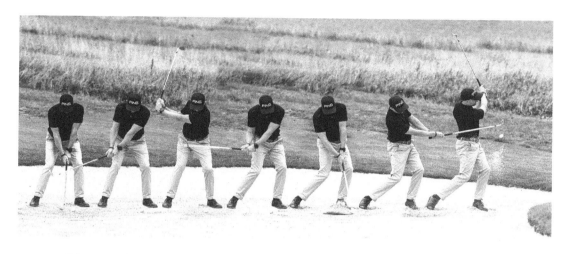

Figure 14 *Greenside bunker set-up and swing sequence*

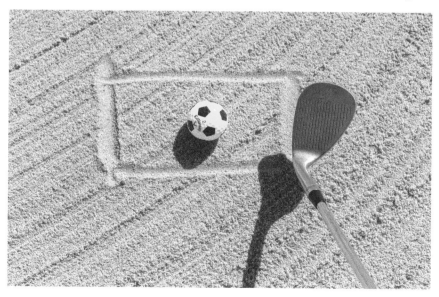

Figure 15
'Dollar bill'
sand shot

I would also recommend an adaptation to the normal grip called the 'butterfly grip'. This requires squeezing the hands slightly closer together – particularly, the bottom hand sitting more on top of the top hand. This positions the hands behind the clubhead and keeps the clubface more open, both of which help you hit the sand first with the bounce and not the leading edge, as Seve did. Theoretically, this is the easiest shot in golf because you don't have to hit the ball; unfortunately, this theory flies out the window, as you'll soon find out!

Swing

Use your longer approach swing as described in Chapter 4. The upper-body turn controls the show again here. Keep your hands and arms relaxed and passive. If you're not gripping the club too tight, the weight and momentum of the club will create the wrist hinge (leverage) automatically. Experiment with the swing length; as long as you're hitting the sand first, you'll make quick progress.

If you are starting to get the ball out consistently, then the next step is to control your distances. The easy way is to keep your backswing the same length and alter the length of your follow-through: short, middle, long. Keeping the point where you hit the sand consistent and only altering the follow-through will adjust the speed through strike and therefore the distance the ball flies out.

Clubface: 'To open or not to open? That is the question'

The SW has 'bounce' (see Figure 16). This refers to the angle at which the sole slopes down from the leading edge to the middle or back of the sole (usually around 10 degrees). This prevents the clubhead from digging too deep into the sand. If the clubhead digs, we have more resistance from the sand and the speed of the clubhead is not transferred efficiently to the ball. In addition, less backspin is imparted to

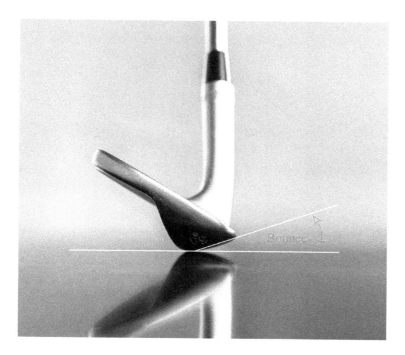

Figure 16

Sand wedge bounce

the ball, making distance control more difficult. When one 'opens up the clubface' (see Figure 15), it is easier to contact the sand first with the bounce as opposed to the leading edge. In addition, the increased loft gives a higher ball flight, also helping the ball to stop quickly on contact with the green. Therefore, when you have the greenside bunker basics under control, experiment with opening the clubface. Two important points: Firstly, open the clubface first and then take your butterfly grip position. You want the clubface to stay open here. If you just twist your wrists or forearms around to open the clubface, you'll shut the clubface again on the downswing. Secondly, open the clubface first and then aim the clubface at your target. The ball will always start where the clubface is aiming; this means your body will be pointing left of target.

Rhythm: Ma-ri-a Jo-se

This mystical character turned up as a tip in a golf magazine I read many years ago. Maria Jose has worked wonders with countless numbers of my students who have tried to muscle the ball out of the bunker instead of swinging rhythmically and letting the bounce do its job. The idea is to say to yourself 'Ma-ri-a' on the backswing and 'Jo-se' on the follow-through.* In any rhythm trick, you are trying to build a coordination of the body parts involved in the swing – in the bunker play, that means coordinating the upper-body turn with the arm swing. Using a name or humming or breathing out give the conscious mind something to do while the subconscious mind gets on with the task in hand –

like singing along to a tune on the radio while you're driving a car. Focusing on rhythm is a powerful way to coordinate an action without thinking too hard. This also works in other areas of the game; however, for whatever reason, Maria Jose seems particularly well-suited to the greenside bunker. I'm sure she will quickly become your bunker buddy!

Fairway bunker

In general, fairway bunkers are positioned a long way back from the green, so we need to make a full swing to send the ball a good distance. Technically, here, we're back to full swing mode. Club choice depends on the lie of the ball and the depth of the bunker. From a good lie in a shallow bunker, it's possible to play a hybrid or fairway wood, while a bad lie (ie part of the ball underneath the level of the sand, making clean contact with the ball virtually impossible) in a deep bunker leaves you with one option – SW and just get the ball out!

You need to make ball contact first. Any contact with the sand before the ball contact will affect the distance, so, unlike the set-up position for greenside bunkers:

- Don't dig your feet in too deep and go under the level of the ball.

- Keep the ball position under the sternum (see Chapter 3).

- Keep grip position normal and grip pressure slightly tighter than normal. (This shortens the muscles in the arms to avoid sand contact. If you overdo it, you'll top the ball.)

Practice: drills and suggestions

Greenside bunker:

- **Hit the line:** With square stance and butterfly grip, hit a line drawn under the sternum without the ball. The aims are to hit the line and 'throw' the sand out of the bunker. When you consistently hit the line, introduce the ball 5 cm ahead of the line. Keep watching the line and not the ball.

- **Hit the line:** As above, with open clubface and stance.

- **Alter distance by altering length of follow-through:** Short follow through, short shot; longer follow-through, longer shot. Always aim 5 cm behind the ball.

Fairway bunker:

- **Full swing:** Experiment with different clubs from different lies. Find out what's sensible and not sensible, possible and impossible.

Bunker HIIT – 10 minutes

- **10 x 12 o'clock to 12 o'clock swing:** With your club or indoor-work stick, take up your posture and butterfly grip face-on to the mirror. Using only your upper-body rotation, allow the stick to swing to 12 o'clock on an imaginary clock face (ie perpendicular to the ground) on both sides of the swing. Keep your lower half stable and upper arms at the sides of your body, as in the posture position. By allowing the club to swing to 12 o'clock, the wrists will hinge as the club swings above the 9 o'clock and 3 o'clock positions. Stand out of your posture after each repetition and renew for the next swing.

- **10 x grip pressure #2:** Repeat the above but focus on keeping the grip pressure constant at #2 (grip pressure #1 is loosest and #5 tightest). Take your hands off the club or stick after each repetition and renew for the next swing.

Golden nuggets

Greenside:

- Ball positioned opposite front foot
- 70% of weight on front foot
- Hands behind clubhead (butterfly grip)
- Dig your feet in
- Fix your eyes on a point 5 cm behind the ball
- Long approach swing
- 'Splash out' the dollar bill

Fairway:

- Don't dig your feet in

- Normal grip – slightly more grip pressure

- Ball under the sternum

- Normal full swing

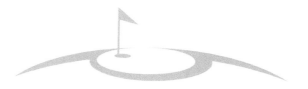

CHAPTER 6

Putting

'This looks like fun... but why is the hole so small?'

On Saturday, 19th July 1980, a Japanese golfer, Isao Aoki, shot 63 strokes around the hallowed links at Muirfield in the third round of the British Open Championship. It was the joint lowest score ever achieved in a major Championship. His score comprised nine 4s and nine 3s, and he took just 24 putts in 18 holes.

The following day, my mum, dad and I were at Muirfield to watch the final round of the Championship. Having watched the highlights on TV the day before, and seen Aoki holing putts from everywhere with the most extraordinary putting style I'd ever seen, I was keen to observe his method live. I headed straight for the practice putting green, and the first thing I noticed when he arrived was that the sweet spot of his golden-headed putter was well worn. Sure, it's the sign of consistent ball striking, but he'd obviously used the same putter for many years. To see that on a putter is remarkable considering the slow swing speed of the putting stroke. I'd never seen that before nor since. And then came his unique putting style: toe of the putter up in the air –

and I mean the club sitting at nearly 45 degrees to the ground! – posture low, hands low. Then, he'd give the ball what can best be described in Scottish terms as 'a wee dunt' – translated as a firm rap, I suppose. And boy, could he putt.

It confirmed to me what I mentioned in Chapter 1: there are many effective styles of full swing, approach play and putting, but this is especially true in putting. So, how do you teach it? Well, there are things that need to happen consistently, whatever the style is. Technically, you need to have good aim and a consistent swing arc to send the ball where you want it to go. Rhythmically, you need to be consistent to get good distance control. Reading the green to visualise the direction in which the ball will roll to the hole is a critical factor. If you get good at all that, you will start to build the most important part of holing putts... belief.

Technique

For simplicity, let's start with a short, straight putt. The first thing to aim is the clubface: 90 degrees to the target line (see Figure 17).

A very important factor to understand in golf swinging technique is that the ball will start out in the direction where the clubface is aiming at strike. If there is no manipulation of the clubface throughout the swing, there's a good chance we can return the clubface to square at the moment of impact and send the ball in the desired direction. Logic. Physics.

We want to make the putting swing as simple and consistent as possible. For this reason, in addition to aiming the clubface we should also aim the body – particularly the shoulders and forearms – and the eyes, parallel to the target line.

Ideal mechanics would have the clubhead swinging straight back and through strike along your target line with the clubface remaining square to the target line throughout the swing. Unfortunately, this is anatomically impossible; there are no straight lines in a golf swing, even by putting – only curves. As we rotate the upper body around the spine from a tilted-upper-body position in golf, the body, hands, arms, pelvis and club will all curve around the spine position. However, in theory, if we start with everything correctly aimed, and make an uncomplicated movement back and through then we have a good chance of returning to our well-aimed position at strike.

So, let's make an uncomplicated movement. Because power is not a requirement in putting, we can simplify the movement we have made with the other swing types. The shoulders control the show here. The feeling to get is that your shoulders tilt up and down in a pendulum motion. Your upper arms stay at the sides of your body, hands and wrists passive. Keep your lower body still – the best putting tip I ever heard was 'Keep your ass still' (just watch the top pros putting for confirmation of that one). In reality, the shoulders are turning, but if you actively try to turn your shoulders, the stroke will likely be too powerful. If the swing is uncomplicated as described, the clubhead should make a consistent arc back and through strike – no manipulation. To check, make a few swings against a wall. The clubhead should curve naturally away from the wall on the backstroke, return to its start position at strike and curve away from the wall again after strike; therefore, the ball position should be at the apex of the arc (see Figure 17).

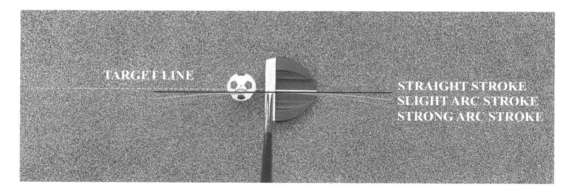

Figure 17 *Clubface aim and swing arcs*

I deliberately haven't talked about putting posture and grip, two of the most critical elements in the full swing and approach shots, until now. That's because they have less influence in putting. You can grip the club in whatever hand and finger position feels comfortable to you;

however, I recommend keeping your shoulders and forearms parallel to your target line, and grip position influences this. Your posture position will influence how the clubhead will curve through the stroke – upright posture will create a sharper curve and a deeper posture position will promote a straighter curve. There is no right or wrong here, but the sharper curve will require a *very* consistent ball position to set the ball off on the desired path.

Rhythm

We've made a good start. Consistent mechanics with as few moving parts as possible is the foundation, but unfortunately it guarantees nothing as far as holing putts is concerned. Next is rhythm, which is essential for developing feel and distance control. I mentioned a 'pendulum motion' of the shoulders, and that is a good way to think about gaining good rhythm. Aim for a feeling that the clubhead speed remains constant whatever the swing length. (Again, feeling and reality are not the same here: in reality, the club accelerates slowly on the backswing, slows down as it changes direction, accelerates through strike and decelerates again as the club reaches its full follow-through – but let's keep it simple!)

To control rhythm, you need to control the grip pressure – any good musician will tell you that. I recommend that you grip the putter as lightly as possible. Particularly on short putts, you want to feel as if the club is almost swinging itself. More important than the amount of pressure is keeping the grip pressure the same until the stroke is complete. As we did for approach play, if you imagine a grip pressure scale of 1–5 where 1 lightest and 5 tightest, we want to be at 1 from start to finish, although 2 would also work. Any more pressure, and your distance control will suffer.

Instinctive distance control

From my experience and research, a large part of neuroscience's aim is to understand and explain what has, until now, been inexplicable. Things you feel or sense intuitively but cannot accurately explain why or how they happen. Often what we call 'gut feeling'. Or everyday actions we consider simple that, when we analyse them, are extremely complicated physical computations.

Imagine sitting bored at work, rolling up a piece of A4 into a ball, and propelling it across the room into the wastepaper basket. The basket-ball equivalent of a 3-pointer from the comfort of your office chair. Did you measure how far you needed to swing your arm back and through? Did you think about what power you needed in your throw to get it to the basket? If you were to throw three sheets of A4 rolled up together, would you need to recalculate the entire throwing process for three times the weight of the original paper ball? Was the distance easier to judge yesterday, when the air conditioning was off and therefore creating less wind resistance, than today? Most people would answer, 'No. I just looked at the paper basket and threw it'. (At this point, the sports psychologist would jump in, put money up front, and ask you to do it again for a hefty bet, therefore changing the mental circumstances. Let's save this for Chapter 7 when we discuss mental preparation.)

This is what I try to explain as 'instinctive putting': look at the hole and react. In reality, you are trying to read the resistance of the grass on the green and the influence of the slope: what does it take to get the ball to the hole, and, if the ball doesn't drop in the hole then I want it to stop at the hole. Fine. But there's one big problem. In golf, you are looking at the ball (AKA the paper ball) and not the hole (AKA the paper basket). We need our eyes to give us the same information as in the paper basket scenario – 'How far?' – but for coordination to the ball we need to look at the ball during the 'throw' (putting stroke) process. In my experience, the solution is as follows:

- Take your aim and set-up position, glancing occasionally at the hole for orientation and general distance surveillance

- When you are ready to play, take one longer look at the hole

- As soon as your eyes are fixed back on the ball, make your stroke

No measurement of swing length, no consideration of power. Just let it happen – 'paper ball and basket' scenario. At the start, this usually requires a leap of faith, but I've seen many players transform their distance control by trusting this process. Instinct. I'm not even going to try and explain it: it just works.

Reading the green

This is a tough one. It would be a lot easier not only if the Scots had invented a bigger ball and bigger hole but also if the greens were always flat. Well, gotta love the challenge. And a twenty-year-old malt whisky is far more complex and enjoyable than a three-year-old one, right? You'll have days when you're great at reading the green and days when you think you'd better pop back to the opticians for a check-up. To me, this is more of an art than a science, and experience and experimentation are more valuable than my words here, but I'll give you a few pointers.

When you're new to golf and are relieved that you've finally reached the green after a few topped and scuffed shots and maybe the odd penalty shot, you delight in the fact that putting is the easiest of all the techniques. Job done... almost. Five putts later, after doubling your score for the hole, you realise you had a false sense of security. So, as well as practising all the aforementioned putting elements, we also need to foresee how the ball is going to roll on the green towards the hole. This is what is meant by 'reading the green' – estimating the effect of slope and green speed on getting the ball close to or into the hole.

Firstly, look for clues even as you approach the green and walk towards your ball. How is the general slope from your ball position to the hole – left side higher than the right, flat, or right side higher than the left?

Secondly, I recommend reading the putt from the hole to the ball – ie backwards – not from the ball to the hole. I usually get funny looks when I mention that to established golfers, but there is method in my madness. Get down low behind your ball relative to the hole – this way, you see the slope of the green in more detail. Note the slope around the hole – this is the zone where the ball will be travelling more slowly (hopefully!) and therefore will be more affected by the slope (eg is the right side of the hole higher than the left side?). This is the main reason why you should read the putt 'backwards'.

After the 'reads', you should be able to visualise where the entry point is. Think of the hole as a clock face and decide where, according to your reading of the green, the ball should enter the clock face; for example, a strong left to right putt enters the hole at 8 o'clock (see Figure 18). While reading, your brain should be building a picture of what you want to happen – how the ball curves towards the entry point of the hole.

If you are uncertain of how much the ball will curve, I guarantee you will hole more putts if you over-read than if you under-read. An under-read putt will never go in the hole; it will just slide by the 'front door'. An over-read putt at a perfect pace can still drop in the 'back door' of the hole.

Once your reading is over, aim your clubface and body in the desired direction to start the putt. I always recommend aiming the clubface first. Trust your aiming instinct here and be confident that the clubface is precisely lined up. Then aim your body and eyes perpendicular to the clubface. One last look at the hole and then let it happen. As I mentioned earlier, no measurement of swing length or strength. Trust your instinct and let it go.

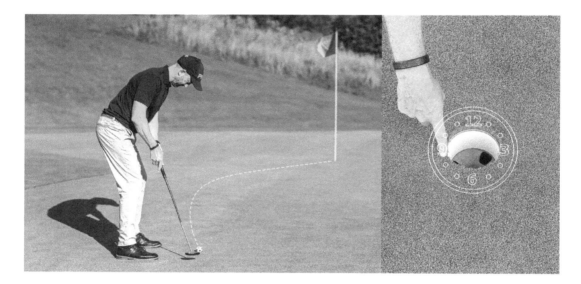

Figure 18 *Reading the green*

There are more complex methods of green reading, which may or may not work for you, but they are outside the scope of this book. In addition, I haven't mentioned 'grain' – the dominant direction in which the grass grows – and its influence on the roll of the ball. That topic is also too complex for this book, and it varies greatly from grass type to grass type and country to country. As ever, read further as you choose, and enjoy the exploration and challenge!

I mentioned at the beginning of this chapter that the most important part of holing putts is belief. I've given you some sound fundamentals which I know can help you become a good, maybe even great, putter, but I've also seen different putting techniques, quite different to how I've described, which work like a charm – Isao Aoki's, for one. My grandfather was the best putter I've ever seen, and he had a very unorthodox style. More so than any of the other disciplines required to play this game, putting can work in many different ways. However, regardless of swing style, what all great putters have in common is that they believe they are going to hole putts. If you don't think the putt is going to go in, it won't, and you should never have attempted success if you believed failure was inevitable.

How, then, do you build belief? Any belief, positive or negative, is a thought that you keep thinking about. You train yourself to believe in something by continually thinking about it, so the sharper your visualisation skills are, seeing the ball dropping in the hole several times in your preparation, the more you are building your belief of holing the putt. This visualisation process also holds true for the full swing or approach play or bunker play, but while their techniques are more complex and the ball is flying rather than rolling along the ground, visualising the perfect shot is more difficult – albeit a great asset – than in putting. By building a reliable putting technique, good rhythm and instinctive distance control, and by 'seeing' how the ball is going to roll into the hole before you send it there, you are building your belief. 'I can do this, and I can see it. Now let it happen' – that's how to putt.

Practice drills and suggestions

- **Technique:** Practise swinging with the toe of the putter head against a wall or club lying on the ground at address. A good pendulum motion from your shoulders will make the clubhead consistently curve away from the wall, back to the wall and away from the wall again, from backswing to downswing.

- **Rhythm:** Give your grip pressure a number of 1 or 2 and hit some putts of varying lengths, ensuring a constant grip pressure from start to finish.

- **Distance control:** Hit five balls from different distances to the same hole, making sure that the time between your last look at the hole and when you start the stroke is 1–2 seconds at most.

- **Reading the green:** From different distances and directions, read the putt and place a coin on the edge or 'clock face' of the hole where you think the ball is going to drop in. Visualise how the ball will curve and roll over the coin. Then make the putt.

Putting HIIT – 15 minutes

If you have carpets or a rug on which a ball will run relatively straight, then you can practise putting. If you have wooden or tiled floors, I recommend you get a putting mat or strip of carpet. Use a putter and real balls and repeat the first three practice drill exercises above. You can also get creative and have some fun putting to small targets: chair legs, over coins, a mug on the floor. I used to do this as a kid, and it made me an awesome putter. I not only believed but expected to hole everything as the target on the golf course was so much bigger than what I'd practised at home.

Golden nuggets

- Precise aim: Clubface first, shoulders and forearms second, eyes third.

- Pendulum motion: Upper arms at your sides, hands passive (grip pressure 1–2), move shoulders in a pendulum movement.

- Rhythm: Keep grip pressure constant from start to finish.

- Instinctive distance control: Trust the information your eyes have given you to judge the pace.

- Green reading: View general slope, read from hole to ball, decide on 'clock face' entry point, visualise the curve, favour over-reading the putt.

- Belief: Build positive belief through 'seeing' the putt holed.

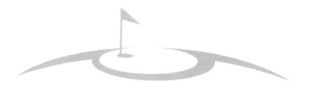

CHAPTER 7

The Golfing Brain

'This game is mental!'

On Sunday, 12 July 1970, at the most famous golf course in the world, the Old Course at St Andrews, Doug Sanders stood over a 30-inch, left to right breaking downhill putt to win his first major, The Open Championship. He had tied for second place in three previous Majors: the USPGA in 1959, the US Open in 1961 and The Open in 1966. Following impressive scores of 68, 71 and 71 in the first three rounds, and getting up and down from the infamous Road Hole bunker at the 17th in the final round, Sanders needed a par 4 at the 358-yard 18th to win by one shot over the greatest player of his time, and indeed all time, Jack Nicklaus.

A prestigious drive left him a 74-yard pitch to the green, over which he presided longer than usual before hitting it over-zealously 35 feet past the flag. A good 'lag' putt left him with the testing 30-incher. A stiff sea breeze was blowing as he addressed the ball, and before starting the putter back he stopped, bent down to remove a blade of grass that had blown onto his line, and immediately readdressed the ball. Four thousand miles away in Fort Worth, Texas, the legendary Ben Hogan leaped out of his chair. 'Walk away, Sanders!' he shouts at his TV screen, 'Walk away!'[16] Sanders didn't walk away. He missed the putt. He also lost the 18-hole play-off the following day to Jack Nicklaus, by one shot.

Golf is difficult and often frustrating. And it is not all under your control – a bad bounce here, an impossible lie there, a gravity-defying brush of the hole with a putt that was sure to go in. It takes a mental toll! And the elements you can control (your swing, your tempo and your thoughts) are often knocked out of kilter by the enormity of a situation – as Doug Sanders found in 1970, when a fairly routine 30-inch putt became a Mental Monster.

How do you prepare mentally to increase your chances of performing at your best, no matter the breaks? There are scores of books on this subject, and I encourage you to read further. But you already know what my approach will be – keep it simple. So, let's talk about the following:

1.   What you can control

2.   What you can't control

3. How to get focused

4. How to find your 'happy'

What you can control

- Your swing: If you're at an early developmental stage, this may be a bit much to ask for. But with practice, your swing should become more consistent and start to function subconsciously. If you are practising as recommended, working on your technique, tempo and routine (see the 'Pre-shot routine' section later in this chapter), then you will be gaining control.

- Your tempo: Tempo often varies between the driving range and the golf course, so practise it and be aware of it on the golf course. 'Am I gripping too tight?' 'Am I swinging too fast?' Get back your control by experimenting with the tempo techniques in Chapter 3.

- Your thoughts: You have full control and choice over what to think. No-one, whatever the situation, can ever take that away from you. People or places or situations may influence you, but you can choose how to react by controlling your thoughts. We'll look at what to practise to help you with this later in this chapter.

What you can't control

This is by no means a comprehensive list, but it will give you the gist:

- Weather

- Bad bounces

- Playing partners (unless you kill them… tempting sometimes, but not recommended)

- The rules

- Distractions (eg noise, animals)

- The golf course

- Par

- The competition (ie how other players perform)

Every round of golf is different. That's all part of the attraction and challenge. The quicker you learn to accept that there are always things in golf that are outside your control, the more patience you will have, and the more you will be able to focus on what you can control. That's how you perform better. In this chapter, I shall introduce the pre-shot routine, an essential tool for focus and shutting out the 'uncontrollables'. I cannot emphasise enough the importance of creating a routine and sticking to it, come what may; it's how you allow yourself to perform at your best. Ben Hogan shouted, 'Walk away, Sanders!' at his TV set to tell Doug Sanders to get back into his routine. Sanders missed a short putt because he was distracted out of his routine by the wind and the situation – both 'uncontrollables'. That missed putt detrimentally affected the rest of his career. He never won a major.

In what I consider to be their most learned and informative book, *Peak Performance*, Magness and Stulberg propose a performance formula:[17]

Performance = Potential – Distractions

For golf, and most other sports:

'Potential' = technical and mental skills, physique and rhythm

'Distractions' = the 'uncontrollables' one must shut out

Simple, right? Yes, in theory. But just as your swing or putting or bunker play requires practice time, so does your mental fitness to perform at your best. You will be influenced by 'the situation' in your forthcoming golfing adventures: 'This 1 metre putt is for par – better take a bit more time over it', or the opposite, 'This 1 metre putt is for a 9 so let's get it quickly over with and go to the next hole'. The physicality of the situation is the same in both cases: a 1 m putt. In both cases, the 1 m putt counts one stroke. When you add all the individual scores for each hole together over the nine or 18 holes, that 1 m putt added one shot, so why treat them so differently? That is what the 'uncontrollable' distraction can do to you. Don't let it!

How to get focused

Here is my recommended mental toolkit.

1. The pre-shot routine

Read this very carefully. This is as important as getting your top-hand grip correct. A good pre-shot routine has the ability to get the above formula really working in your favour ie great Performance by allowing your Potential to play great shots and simultaneously cutting out all Distractions (the 'uncontrollables'). Before we get into the details, it's important that you develop your own routine that (a) gets you in your comfort zone and (b) doesn't take too long, not only because that is bad etiquette (see Chapter 9 on etiquette and rules) but also because of your focus time. Here's an example and I'll discuss the important points afterwards before you experiment on the driving range and course with your own routine.

Example for a pre-shot routine:

> *Distance to flag*: 110 m
> *Lie*: fairway/good

Wind direction and strength: left to right, moderate

Green: hard and fast

Let's say your normal 110 m shot is an 8 iron. Because the green is hard and fast, you choose a 9 iron and decide to land the ball short of the flag and aim 5 m left to account for the wind. You visualise how the shot will fly to the target. Your decisions on all the conditions are now complete.

You take a practice swing to feel good rhythm. You aim up left of the flag, look at the target, return your eyes to the ball and make a nice rhythmic swing. Job done.

Regardless of the result, you have focussed from start to finish on the processes you can control: swing, tempo, thoughts. Whatever the shot, whatever the difficulty, whatever the situation, that is all you can ever do. Don't let the uncontrollables dictate anything else. And if you're thinking what I'm thinking, you're right – that doesn't just apply to golf.

Let's look at the important factors here:

- **Decision-making:** How's the lie? Which club to use? How will the conditions (lie, wind, etc) affect the shot?

- **Visualisation:** What do you want to happen – the end result, the ball flight?

- **Feel:** How should the swing feel to get you the desired result? Make a practice swing.

- **Let go:** Aim, set-up, go!

Let me expand a little.

Hopefully, the **decision-making** process is clear and dependent on your level of play and expectation for your own performance.

Visualisation is key. It's difficult to perform any task successfully if you can't see what the outcome will be. And your outcome needs to be what you want (eg 'I want the ball to fly high and straight and land next to the flag'). If you want to avoid the water hazard, then I'm afraid you've programmed 'water hazard' into your subconscious visualisation process and have a good chance of landing in the water hazard. Do not underestimate the power of the subconscious, and be careful what you think about; you'll attract it.

Feel: Experiment with practice swings. If they don't add to your confidence, don't make one, especially if it only brings doubt (eg 'That was a poor practice swing, but I'll go ahead anyway'). If practice swings help you feel good rhythm or confirm good technique, then do them. But don't do too many, for two reasons: firstly, it's poor etiquette – takes too much time; and secondly, you're wasting precious energy. If you make on average 50 full swing shots in a round, and make two practice swings per shot, then you're making 150 full swings per round.

That can also be a strain on the small muscles and joints of the lower arm which are most prone to injury in the golf swing, leading to tendonitis or tennis or golfer's elbow.

Let go: It's easy to say, but try and give up control and let what you've practised take over. Often, that means giving the conscious mind something to do so that the subconscious can perform the task alone. Let's take the analogy of walking 100 m down a sidewalk which is 1 m wide. Usually, you can perform this task while thinking of other things, such as how hungry you are, who you're going to meet, the last text you received or your plan for tomorrow. Then, you're given a bet: walk the same 100 m down the sidewalk, and if you don't fall off it you win $1 million. You'd then concentrate fully on every step and may be walking a bit unnaturally. Then, for $2 million, you're given the same 100 m sidewalk challenge but it's 1,000 feet up in the air and the sidewalk is made of glass. Physically, the task hasn't changed, but the uncontrollables have. Just think about how hungry you are again, and you've got this! – ie give the conscious mind something to do, and let your incredibly clever subconscious take over.

2. Mental tricks to help let go

So, let me give you some suggestions for occupying the conscious mind and letting your subconscious control the show. The first three I mentioned briefly in Chapter 3, but let's look at them in a bit more detail.

1. **Breathing:** You should be good at this if you're still alive, right? So focus on your breathing as you swing. Breathing out during the downswing is most likely to give you a relaxed, rhythmic swing; therefore, either breathe in on the backswing and out on the downswing or breathe out the entire swing. Practising this can help let the subconscious take over and give you good rhythm.

2. **Grip pressure:** Recall our grip pressure scale of 1–5, where 1 is lightest and 5 is tightest, and hold the club with grip pressure 3. More important than the pressure level is that it remains the same from start to finish. Hit a few balls and ask yourself at the end of each swing, 'Is my grip pressure still at 3?' If not, where did it change – during the takeaway, backswing or transition? You are building an awareness of the pressure, which affects the rhythm. In addition, you are occupying the conscious mind and letting the subconscious get on with the swing. You may be amazed at how well you hit the ball when your grip pressure remains relaxed and constant.

3. **Centring:** This is a little more difficult but potentially a very effective focus to allow the body to perform a balanced, efficient and powerful movement. In Tai Chi, learning to originate all your moves from the Dantian or tan t'ien – the physical centre – is an important grounding force. It is seen as a reservoir of energy located about two inches below the navel in the middle of your body.[18] When you can focus your thoughts on this point

during an entire golf swing, it's more than a trick to occupy the conscious mind. It improves balance, stability and power – as in Tai Chi, working the power from the inside outwards. This takes practice, and I encourage all my students to take part in yoga or Pilates to strengthen this awareness (along with all the other benefits of core strength, stability and breathing that these disciplines bring). It may be the greatest focus you can take with you onto the golf course.

If you watched rugby in the late 1990s and early 2000s, you may have seen the extraordinary kicking feats of the Englishman Jonny Wilkinson. This was centring at its most visible in a sporting context. When kicking for goal between the posts, Wilkinson would get into a part-crouched position, clasping his hands together and looking repeatedly up from the ball to the posts, visualising his intention. He was also focussing into his centre to calm his mind and ready his body for the powerful, balanced, precise motion to come.

4. **Humming:** This is simple but effective, although you might get some funny looks. As with grip pressure, the goal here is to hum at a constant tone throughout the swing. The first few attempts, your humming tone will rapidly become high pitched as you come into the strike – like a motorbike revving its engine or a wasp getting irritated that it can't fly out of the window. With practice, you will calm the inner 'wasp'.

Your pre-shot routine gets you into the 'zone'. It's no mystery; it's just you, visualising what you want, focussing on what you can control and 'letting go' in the active phase by giving the conscious mind an effective task that's disconnected from complex or technical thoughts. The key words here are 'want', 'visualisation' and 'focus'.

3. Practising positivity and focus

It's not often you see a miserable pessimist winning golf tournaments – or, for that matter, becoming a successful businessperson or performing artist. From my basic understanding of physiology and neuroscience, thoughts control your body chemistry, which in turn control your mood and performance. I also hold the well supported belief that you attract to you what you think about; increasing evidence from quantum physics and epigenetics supports this 'gut feeling' theory.[19] I've experienced it in the world of golf a thousand times – a gut feeling that I'm going to miss a short putt almost guarantees the negative outcome, while if I have a good gut feeling about holing the putt I often do. Frankly, I don't give a rat's about whether the theory can be scientifically proven or not – I just imagine hitting the fairway, landing on the green and holing the putt. Water hazard? What water hazard!

As with practising your full swing or short game, the mind needs to be trained to make this positive mindset a habit. I recommend practising trying to see the positive in every situation, person and thing. Let's say you have a work colleague who annoys you. You can't stand to be in their presence and dread going into work when you know they will be there. Ask yourself, 'Is there one positive thing I can find about this person, however banal it may be?' Do they always wear nice socks? Do you love the way they style their hair or always wear nice suits? This may sound weird, but let's think about what's happening here. You are changing your thoughts. Your brain chemistry is changing because you're focussed on something positive. Your mood and performance have changed because of your positive chemistry. Is that person likely to respond differently to you because suddenly you're in a positive mood, when previously you were always in a negative mood in their company? For sure! Changing a potential negative on the golf course, for example, 'Oh no, I always hit it in that water hazard', into a positive, 'I'll use the water hazard to help show me where I should be aiming', can, with a little practice, have the same mood changing and performance enhancing effect.

So much for positivity; what about focus? Holding your concentration over 3 or 4 hours on a round of golf can be difficult. I have two pieces of advice for you here. Firstly, you only need to concentrate when you're preparing for and playing your shot. At all other times try and switch off. Keep your eyes above the horizon, watch the birds, smell the flowers, chat with your partner or whatever works. Don't dwell on the past (eg your score or previous shots) or in the future (eg your potential score or the difficulty of the next hole). Secondly, maintain total focus on your pre-shot routine to avoid distractions. My two tips for practising and improving your focus are mindfulness and meditation. There is often overlap between these two terms, but I'll keep my take on their practical application related to golf.

Mindfulness involves bringing your attention to experiences happening in the present moment, particularly those relating to your body. This requires focussing on a specific body part with no judgement as to what is happening with it. If I, as your guide, told you to be aware of what's happening with your right foot during the golf swing, you would hit a few balls and tell me afterwards what your right foot did, such as how the weight moved there in the backswing, how the sole stayed flat on the ground till shortly before impact, and how it then released the weight and ended with the heel off the ground.

This is awareness of what is happening in your body in the present moment, and it can dramatically affect your ability to improve a swing movement. If you can't feel the bad movement, you will find it almost impossible to change to a new movement. One of the key elements of making a swing change is feeling the difference between the old and the new. Practising body awareness is enormously helpful in this respect.

Additionally, I mentioned switching off between shots. Here, awareness of your environment can help you stay in the present. The great Sam Snead, American pro golfer and 82-time PGA Tour winner in the 1940s and 1950s, was not joking or belittling the importance of mentally switching off when he said, 'Between shots, I smell the flowers.' This was mindfulness in action before anybody knew what mindfulness meant. If you are struggling to stay in the moment between shots, you can also focus on your walking – the way the weight changes in your feet from heels to toes, how the muscles in your legs work and then switch off, how the ground feels beneath your feet. The aim is to quiet the mind, stay in the present, avoid unnecessary distractions, and allow the deliberate concentration to start more easily when it is time to prepare for the next shot.

Meditation involves achieving a physical and psychological calm through focussing the mind. This requires a longer period of quiet contemplation than mindfulness. I suggest finding a quiet place, ideally for 10–40 minutes. Often, the focus is on the breath for the entire duration of the meditation, and counting breaths is also a common practice to increase awareness or dampen distraction. Initially during meditations, thoughts will often drift away from the breath. The trick is not to judge your poor focus but be aware that it has drifted, accept it, congratulate yourself for noticing it, and return to your focus on the breath. This takes practice and I recommend starting with 10 minutes a day. Put a timer on and do it sitting up rather than lying down if you might otherwise fall asleep, and there are many phone apps which will guide you through a basic meditation. There's nothing complicated, mystical or religious about it; just find a little time each day, ideally not long after you awake in the morning when the brain is still 'quiet'. Relax and enjoy it.

How to find your 'happy'

There are many well-documented benefits to meditation, including reducing stress, improving brain function and gaining a calmer persona. From a golfing perspective, meditation assists in clarity of decision-making, shot visualisation, body feeling, keeping calm under pressure, reducing negative reaction to poor shots and eliminating distractions. In my experience, the positive effects of meditation often go unnoticed in the heat of the battle on the golf course; however, on analysis of your round you will start to notice how you didn't react negatively to a bad shot, or that your playing partners' constant chatter or the wind or the rain didn't disturb you. You will notice that you're enjoying your golf more, no matter the score, because you're calm and positive. The happy chemicals are flowing! It might just change your life in a positive way too.

I find my 'happy' on the golf course by marvelling at and appreciating the beautiful nature that abounds in most golfing environments the world over. It really is a privilege to play this challenging sport in such magnificent and variable surroundings – the birdlife, beautiful trees, wildflowers, butterflies, and more. And in between shots we have the time to observe, appreciate and switch off. Your performance will vary from day to day, hole to hole and even shot to shot, but there will always be something to marvel at and bring you back to your happy place. Great performances can emanate from this state.

Practice drills and suggestions

Build your pre-shot routine. Play different shots with different clubs, lengths and targets, and experiment to find what routine works best for you. The routine should include the following elements:

- What do you want to happen?

- Visualise a positive outcome.

- Make a practice swing to feel how that positive outcome will happen.

- Address the ball and let it happen (combining the 'let go' trick and picturing your positive outcome).

Mental HIIT – 10 minutes

It's possible to do all of these exercises in a day, but you can schedule them as you please.

1. **Mindfulness:** You can do this anywhere. Bring your awareness to different body parts; for example, start at the top of your head and describe to yourself what you feel, then move down to the muscles around your eyes, then to your ears, mouth, neck and further down. You can start anywhere and go anywhere. The key is to stay focussed on your body and relay what you feel

to yourself without any judgement. If you find this difficult to do for 10 minutes and notice that your mind wanders off, start with 2 minutes and build up.

2. **Meditation:** Find a quiet place where you won't be disturbed and put on a timer for 10 minutes. Close your eyes and focus on your breathing. Try to breathe in through your nose, allowing your stomach to expand, and breathe out through your mouth. It helps at the start to count your breaths. Try and do 30 cycles (1 cycle = breathe in + breathe out). Initially, your mind may wander to other thoughts; that's fine, just notice it and return your thoughts to your breathing. With practice, you can increase the number of cycles or just forget counting and set your timer for however long you like.

3. **Visualisation:** You can start this exercise once you have done some practising and have hopefully seen videos of your good shots, or you've watched other good golfers at the driving range or on TV or YouTube. Find a quiet place where you won't be disturbed for 10 minutes. Sit and close your eyes and try to visualise yourself making swings or approaches or putts with successful outcomes. For a full swing, you may visualise your pre-shot routine, your swing, the ball flight, where the ball lands and where it finishes, always hitting fairways and always ending close to the flag.

Golden nuggets

☞ Controllables: Focus on what you can control: swing, tempo, thoughts

☞ Pre-shot routine: Decide what you want, visualise it, feel it (practice swing) and let it happen

☞ Let it happen: Breathing, grip pressure, centring, humming

☞ Practise positivity: Find the positives in everyday situations

☞ Focus: Experiment with mindfulness and meditation to improve your concentration, clarity of thought and calmness

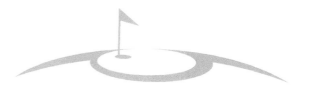

CHAPTER 8

Fit For Golf

'OK, I realise now that golf is a sport. Do I need to get fit?'

When I was 46 years old, I decided I wanted to try and play on the Seniors Tour and, specifically, to qualify for the British Seniors Open when I turned 50: golf's qualifying age for 'Senior' status. I had tried to qualify for the British Open on three previous occasions, all unsuccessfully, and the frustrated golfer within me saw a fresh opportunity. I still had a great short game, but I decided I needed to change everything if I was to succeed: swing, mental approach and fitness.

During this time, I worked with a business and sports psychologist, Frank Troetschkes, who had notably worked with Switzerland's former tennis star, Michel Kratochvil ATP 35. We had some great sessions together and I carry some of his sound advice to this day. After one of our early sessions, he said to me, 'Is there anything physically that stands in your way of getting to the level you want?' I mentioned a potential arthritic problem in the third finger of my right hand. 'Ah, I heard of a great remedy for arthritis when I was in South Africa. You get white sultanas, gotta be the white ones. You put them in a jar, fill the jar up with gin, leave them in the fridge for a week and then eat a few every day.' I replied, 'Wow, does that really work?' to which, without hesitation, he quipped, 'Does it matter?'

While there may or may not be magic remedies for bodily ailments, there are certainly no lotions, potions or pills for body fitness. We are designed as hunter-gatherers. Only sitting on our arses for hours, eating and sleeping is not what we are designed to do and will almost certainly result in a multitude of health problems.

I decided early in my project to work towards the Seniors Tour that I would have some advantage over the 'oldies' if I took care of my body and so began my journey into golf fitness. I am privileged to have worked with many learned people in the past eight years, including: Daniel Huser and Christian Meissgeier from Physio Puma, who worked with the Swiss national football team; the late great Ramsay McMaster, golf physiotherapist, who worked with many top golf pros, including Jason Day and Henrik Stenson; Michael Dalgleish, internationally respected authority in golf-specific physiotherapy; REHA Klinik Rheinfelden, who specialise in golf injury prevention and treatment; CorpoSana Fitness and Health Centre, who looked after the great Roger Federer early in his career; and golf biomechanics expert Jean-Jacques Rivet, who has worked with Lydia Ko and Justin Rose. So now, I'm not only a pretty fit 'senior', but I also have a good base understanding of golf-specific injuries and training. I work out at home 3–5 times per week, attend yoga class once a week and have experimented with CrossFit. I haven't qualified for the British Seniors Open yet, but the journey continues and I'm injury-free and full of energy!

You can take your golf fitness as far as you like, but the order in level of importance and training commitment is:

1. Avoid getting injured

2. Have good mobility to make an efficient and powerful movement

3. Have balance and stability to build a consistent movement

4. Build power and speed for distance

While the pros will be working at all four levels, in this book I shall concentrate only on injury prevention and mobility. If you get the fitness bug, then get a good trainer who understands the golf swing and go for balance, stability and power – muscle up to bomb it!

HIIT – 15 minutes

Personally, and I think I speak for many of us, the thought of exercising for more than 15 minutes doesn't get me excited. I know that it will be beneficial and that I will enjoy the results – but enjoyment? Nope. So, once more, I'm going to keep this super simple. I know this 15-minute routine works because I do it every morning.

Injury prevention and mobility exercises

1. Blackroll® – 7 minutes

    Blackroll® is a solid foam roll available at fitness stores. It has several functions: it improves flexibility, mobility and muscle performance, prevents muscle pain, improves blood circulation, and improves posture to maintain good body form during workouts. I recommend purchasing a Blackroll®. Pop onto YouTube, type in 'Blackroll® exercises' and get started. The videos will be more helpful to you than me showing a series of pictures. There is also informative medical advice on their website, www.blackroll.com.

2. Mobility (GOWOD app) – 8 minutes

    There are many mobility apps, but I find GOWOD, aimed at CrossFit athletes but applicable for all, brilliant. There is a daily protocol which gives you a different 8-minute stretching sequence each day to avoid neglecting any part of the body. The exercise videos and explanations are great, too.

That's it! Didn't I say it was simple? It's also effective. Having good mobility is key for the golf swing, and the less chance you have of getting muscle strains, the longer you can practise. I do 15 minutes of meditation and the above routine each morning before breakfast – a healthy, productive and beneficial start to the day.

Golden nuggets

Start your day with 7 minutes of Blackroll and 8 minutes of mobility stretches to:

- Avoid injury

- Reduce your limitations for swinging the golf club powerfully and efficiently

- Increase your ability to practise for longer periods

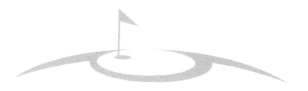

CHAPTER 9

'FORE!' – Etiquette And Rules

I came to work in Switzerland in 2003 and made my first visit as a spectator to the European Tour Event, the Omega Masters at Crans Montana, in 2005. I was standing next to the tee at the long par-5 9th following the Englishman Barry Lane and the Italian Emanuele Canonica. I'd heard the latter's diminutive stature hid an unbelievably powerful swing, and I was looking forward to seeing it in action. He teed the ball up, made an innocuous practice swish and set up to the ball. As he glanced to his proposed landing point, a photographer meandered into the fairway at about 300 yards, kneeled down and pointed his lens back to the tee, presumably to photograph the oncoming drive. Canonica stood back from his ball. His caddie, a hardened, old-school, no-beating-about-the-bush Scotsman, was incensed at the photographer. He hastily took a few strides forward and started bawling expletives and waving furiously at the wrongdoer, intending to send him back to the rough, out of the way of Canonica's expected bullet. The crowd and the two patient pros had a chuckle at the colourful language as the photographer held up an apologetic hand and scuffled back into the rough. The caddie turned back to his player and, in a thick Glaswegian accent, said, 'Awright, boss, pick a line and hit it'. Canonica readdressed the ball, picked his line and let loose a swing with enough ferocity to slay a charging grizzly bear. The ball fizzed off and whistled like a rocket, landed where the photographer had knelt at about 300 yards, and ran on another 50 yards. The crowd gasped and then applauded enthusiastically. Barry Lane exclaimed, 'And **** did he hit it!'

There will always be distractions in this game – weather, animals, insects, sudden noises, etc – as it's played in a wild and uncontrollable environment. That's part of the charm. But distractions shouldn't come from your playing partners, other golfers, or bystanders who know and practise good golf course etiquette. Respect for your fellow golfers is just one part of course etiquette, and the photographer should have known that. He would also have learned quickly, if he'd stayed where he was, that golf can be a dangerous game! Golf etiquette is not outdated, fuddy-duddy, airs-and-graces, upper-class established, social and political correctness. It is:

1. **Respect for your fellow golfers:** Playing safely and remaining quiet and still during play to let them concentrate

2. **Respect for the golf course:** Leaving it in the condition in which you would wish to find it

3. **Pace of play:** Playing at a tempo which doesn't impede the enjoyment for you, your playing partners or others playing the golf course

Some say that golf has too many rules. I disagree. The little ball finds itself in an incredible number of situations in this 'wild' environment, and we need rules that cover each one; otherwise, we'd have to make the field of play more limited and unnatural, and that should never be the goal. It is not necessary to know all the rules off by heart. Even as an official Rules Referee, I didn't know them all, but I knew where to find them in the official rules book if challenged. In this book, I will stick to covering the situations that occur most often since you should know these off by heart. For further reading, please consult the bibliography at the back of this book.

Let's kick off with good etiquette and afterwards discuss the frequently occurring rules situations.

Etiquette

Safety and respect for your fellow golfers

Both the golf club and the ball can be dangerous weapons. Many serious injuries have occurred on golf courses and driving ranges from a club being swung without due regard for people standing nearby, or from a ball travelling at great speed. Thankfully, in all the years I've been playing I have only been struck once by a golf ball. It was at Looe Golf Club in Cornwall. I was standing in the fairway when a ball from the next tee veered violently left, flew over the rough separating our holes, took one bounce and struck me hard in the left hip. I went down like a sack of potatoes, letting out a bloodcurdling wail as I hit the deck. My partners thought I'd been shot! After my amateur dramatics and letting down my trousers to inspect the damage – probably not good etiquette in itself – I found that I was badly bruised but still able to play on. It made me realise, however, what damage could have been done if the ball had struck me in the head, especially if it hadn't bounced.

Unfortunately, the player who struck this shot did not shout 'FORE!' – golf's warning word that a ball is flying in an unintended direction towards another player or players. Whether I would have had time to react or not is another matter as the ball was travelling so fast, but shouting 'FORE' as quickly and as loudly as possible on realisation that your ball could endanger someone is good etiquette and potentially important in preventing injury. (N.B. Check your insurance policy for third-party liability and purchase additional golf cover if necessary.) If you are playing and hear the shout 'FORE!', take action: immediately cover your head with your arms and crouch down to make yourself a smaller target.

One of the most well-known, successful and charismatic golfers of the 1970s was the Mexican Lee Trevino. He is held in the same high regard as other greats of the time – Nicklaus, Player, Palmer, Watson. However, I recall a story from my time as the head pro at Panmure GC in Angus, Scotland, when Trevino's name was used with disdain in circumstances entirely unconnected to the great Mexican.

The 14th hole at Panmure is a par 5 with 'out of bounds' and the main Dundee-to-Aberdeen railway line running all the way down the right side. It was a Saturday Medal competition, and one of our most charismatic members (fondly nicknamed 'the Aerosol' because he used to spray golf balls all over the place) teed the ball up on the 14th and was ready to launch another unpredictable missile. On the railway line about 150 yards from the tee was a stationary inspection truck – an open wagon that was engineless and manually operated with a lever that a person on each side would push down like a seesaw to get the truck in motion. The two workers on board, inspecting the track, were oblivious to the erratic golfer on the tee. The Aerosol let fly and the ball sliced off to the right at great speed – 'FORE!' The ball struck the wagon and pinged back and forth off the metal lever, the truck floor, the railway line and the stones. The two workers leaped from the wagon and took cover, not knowing what had happened. As the hubbub died down, one of the workers looked back to the tee and realised that the ball must have come from the Aerosol, who, to the workman's horror, was preparing to hit a second ball. 'Look out,' he cried to his workmate. 'That f*****g Trevino's teeing up anither wan!'

Golf, as you may already have realised, demands concentration. While outside noise and distraction from wind, birds or planes is uncontrollable, noise and distraction from your playing partners is unacceptable. In the name of fair play, you should remain quiet and still when your playing partners are preparing for and playing their shots. This includes whispering (often more annoying than talking), jangling tees and coins in your pocket (infuriating) and ripping the Velcro® to open your glove (punishable by death).

Respect for and repair of the golf course

As with most points of etiquette and rules, care for the golf course is common sense. If you damage something with your club, ball or cart, you must repair it to allow following golfers to enjoy their game, as golfers playing in front of you have also done for you. The main damage-and-repair requests are:

1. Replace your divots on the fairway and rough

2. Repair your pitch marks on the greens

3. Rake over your footprints in the bunkers

4.   Repair spike marks on the green

5.   Keep carts away from the teeing ground and greens

On occasion, I'll hear a golfer comment on the above tasks, 'That's the greenkeeper's job'. Well, the greenkeeper and his team have usually an area of 100–200 acres (40–80 hectares) to attend to on a normal 18-hole golf course. That is at least 19 greens (including the practice green) that need mowing daily and holes changed two or three times weekly, and that require regular treatments of sanding and aeration, as well as 18 fairways and a driving range that need cutting two to three times weekly. There's also a semi-rough that needs cutting once a week, bunkers that need raking daily and their edges trimmed weekly, and gardens around the clubhouse and car park that need regular attention, not to mention maintenance of the drainage and irrigation systems, planting and maintenance of trees, upkeep of pathways, rubbish collection and driving range ball collection. And they have to do all this work in a stop-start manner because there are golfers at all times of day on the area that they endeavour to maintain in immaculate condition for all to enjoy. So, do you think the greenkeeper has the time or inclination to repair every lazy, arrogant, ignorant golfer's divot or pitch mark? Would it be OK if I came around to your house, walked through your flowerbeds and then said, 'Hey, it's your garden, you fix it'? No! (Phew, rant over.) Thank you in advance for your care and consideration for the golf course.

Now that we've touched and dealt with that nerve, let's move on to the third part of golfing etiquette:

Pace of play

How long should a game of golf take? If you're talking about a busy resort course, with groups of four playing every 10 minutes, 18 holes in 4 to 4 1/2 hours is fine, as long as it doesn't impede the enjoyment of your playing partners or others playing the golf course. If you are two people, playing a 9-hole golf course in the middle of nowhere with no-one else on it, nobody will give a hoot whether you play it in 1 hour or 7 hours. It's all about everyone enjoying the game on the beautiful playing field.

However, I know from painful experience how unenjoyable golf can be when you are waiting to hit every shot and remain on the golf course for 5 to 6 hours. Flow keeps the game going, so let's talk about what enhances or impedes flow.

'Faff: to spend time in ineffectual activity.'[20]

I must highlight this brilliantly descriptive word here. It is the main reason for slow play on the golf course. Over many years, I have come to realise that slow play has little to do with playing ability, walking pace, rules knowledge, experience or age and everything to do with faffing about. In his brilliantly clear and concise book, *Golf Etiquette*

Quick Reference: A Golfer's Guide to Correct Conduct, Yves C Ton-That lists the ten golden rules for playing at a good tempo.[21] I list them here and give my own brief explanations. Next to each one I could add, 'Don't faff about!'

1. **Be ready to play:** This is rightly number one on the list and the major theme in slow play. Let's say that it's my turn to play from the tee but I'm not ready yet – I haven't got my glove on, my ball and tee peg aren't in my hand, and I haven't chosen my club yet. Tick, tick, tick. It takes me 20 seconds to get myself ready. I take three practice swings – another 20 seconds. Tick, tick, tick. I set up to the ball, studying everything I have to do – grip, alignment, visualise, relax – another 20 seconds. Tick, tick, tick. I eventually hit the ball, but it's taken me up to a minute longer to play than if I was prepared to play, took one practice swing and had an efficient routine. Let's say this faffing about takes place at the teeing ground on all 18 holes – that's 18 minutes lost to my faffing. And what if I did that on every full shot? I'd be responsible for over an hour's delay! Intolerable and so easily solved. Just be aware of when it is your turn to play or if you can play safely without delay – what is now referred to as 'ready golf' – then do so. This awareness alone could solve all slow play problems at busy courses all over the world.

2. **Take your equipment with you:** Sounds logical, but you'd be surprised how many people leave the bag 10 metres behind

their ball, walk forward, play their shot, walk back and collect it. Tick, tick, tick. Faff, faff, faff.

3. **Only one practice swing:** For the sake of good playing tempo and to conserve your energy on the golf course, take only one practice swing.

4. **Watch the ball:** Another pet hate of mine is hearing, 'Where is my ball?' Follow your ball flight (and those of your playing partners) till it drops. If you think your ball may be difficult to find, pick a mark near where the ball should be (eg a bush or tree), then proceed to the next step.

5. **Play a provisional ball:** It takes a few seconds to hit a second ball if you think your first may be lost, but if you don't find your first one you'll be able to carry on with the provisional ball (see the rule on provisional balls in the next section).

6. **Keep your position:** Start times vary from club to club but are usually every 10 minutes. That's enough time to play a par 3 hole and most par 4s. That means, if you are keeping your position on the golf course, the group ahead of you is never much more than one hole in front of you. Regardless of the actual time it takes to play 18 holes, if you keep this pace no-one has the right to complain about your speed. If you lose this gap on the flight in front and the group behind is starting to wait for you:

7. **Allow faster players to play through:** Ideally at the start of the next hole. Your group play their tee shots then invite the faster group to play through on completion of the previous hole. The faster group play their tee shots, and you all walk forward together. When they play their next shots and are safely far enough forward, you can continue to play.

8. **Pick your ball up:** Outside of when you are playing under Competition rules, I recommend you pick up your ball (ie finish the hole and go to the next tee) once you are 4 over par for the hole and still not near holing out.

9. **Finish off short putts:** If the ball finishes within a few centimetres of the hole and you can easily finish off without standing on anybody else's line of putt, tap it in. It saves a lot of time marking, waiting, replacing and holing out.

10. **Leave the green:** All discussions and marking the scorecard on completion of the hole should take place on the way to or on the next teeing ground.

If you are playing safely, repairing the course as you go and playing at a good tempo, you, your playing partners, and the groups playing behind you will be relaxed and enjoying their time playing golf. This is how the game is meant to be played. If you only know a handful of rules about how to play the game but practise good etiquette, you will be a credit to the game and loved by all in the golfing community for it.

Common rules situations

There are thirty-four golfing rules, all with numerous subsections, and four appendices. If you suffer from insomnia, I suggest that you read the official rules book and, if that's not enough to send you into the land of Nod, get a copy of *Decisions on the Rules of Golf* – it's melatonin in print form. Seriously, though, these are two necessary books to explain the procedures for all playing conditions and situations, in very precise language so as to avoid misinterpretation. Thankfully, you don't have to know them all. I recommend getting Yves C Ton-That's *Golf Rules* Quick Reference 2019 or download his Expert Golf - iGolfrules app for quick reference on the round if you are unsure of the procedure.[22] Additionally, golf's ruling body, the Royal and Ancient Golf Club of St Andrews (R&A), produces a simplified Player's Edition of the Rules of Golf.

To help you understand how to play by the rules and improve your pace of play by knowing the most commonly used rules situations, I explain a few as they would occur on playing a golf hole – from teeing ground to holing out (see Figure 19).[23]

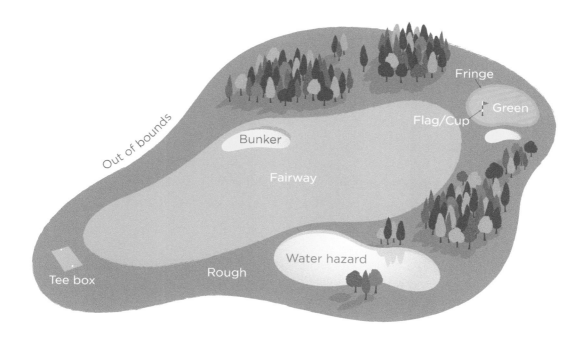

Figure 19 *Golf course rules terminology*

Definition of a stroke: A stroke is the forward movement of the club made with the intention of striking at and moving the ball. If no contact with the ball is made but the intent was to strike it, it counts as one stroke (ie air shots count).

Teeing ground: Your ball may be placed on or teed up on the teeing ground – an area defined by markers and up to two club lengths deep.

Out of bounds: If your ball, played from the tee or any other position on the course, goes over the limit defined by white posts, your ball is out of bounds. You must immediately play another ball from the same point and add 1 penalty shot.

Ball lost: If you are unable to find your ball within 3 minutes of searching, the ball is lost. You must play another ball from the last position and add 1 penalty shot.

Provisional ball: To maintain good pace of play, if you think your ball may be either out of bounds or difficult to find, immediately play another ball from the same position, declaring to your partners that it is a 'provisional ball'. This means that, on the provision that the last ball is out or lost, you will continue with this ball with the addition of 1 penalty stroke. On the teeing ground, you may tee the provisional ball; outside the teeing ground, you must drop the ball.

Dropping a ball: A ball to be dropped must be dropped from knee height not nearer to the hole than the previous shot or where the ball entered a penalty area (see the penalty area rule).

Ball played as it lies: Your ball must be played as it lies and you are not allowed to improve the lie of the ball in any way (eg by flattening the grass behind the ball).

Ball unplayable: If you deem the ball to be unplayable, you may, under penalty of 1 shot,

- Drop the ball within two club lengths of where it lies, not nearer to the hole, or

- On an extension of the line from the flag through the current ball position, or

- Replay from the previous position

Ball at rest moved: If you address the ball anywhere outside the teeing ground or the green and the ball moves, you are penalised 1 shot and must return the ball to its original position. This can often occur when the ball lies in the rough, so to avoid a penalty do not place your club-head on the ground behind the ball in such circumstances.

Loose impediments: These are any natural objects not either fixed or growing (loose leaves, twigs, etc). All loose impediments may be removed before play providing that the ball does not move. If the ball moves, you are penalised 1 shot and the ball must be replaced.

Obstructions: These are any unnatural objects within the boundary of the golf course, but not including unnatural objects defining out of bounds, eg white posts or fences.

Movable obstructions: These include a marker post or rubbish bin; they may be temporarily moved if, for example, the stance or swing is impeded, and replaced after the shot.

Immovable obstructions: These include artificial paths or roads. You may take a penalty-free drop by determining the nearest point of relief – where you have free stance and swing – not nearer the hole, measuring an additional club length from this point, and dropping the ball from knee height within the club length.

Penalty areas: These are marked by red or yellow posts on the golf course. If your ball is playable, you may play it without penalty. If the ball is unplayable or lost in the penalty area (eg in a water hazard), you may drop another ball outside the penalty area under penalty of one stroke.

Bunker: The bunker is the only location where you are not allowed to ground your club behind the ball in the address position as it would likely improve the lie of the ball (penalty 1 shot). If you deem the ball unplayable in the bunker, you may, under penalty of 1 stroke, drop the ball in the bunker either within two club lengths, not nearer to the hole from where it lies, or on an extension of the line from the flag through the ball. You may also drop a ball on an extension of this line outside the bunker but under penalty of 2 shots.

Green: The green is the only location where you are allowed to mark and clean your ball during play of a hole. Always mark the ball's position with a coin or similar behind the ball in relation to the hole. Always replace the ball in exactly the same spot. You may remove loose impediments and repair pitch marks, old holes and spike marks on your line of play. You are allowed to hit the flagstick when it is standing upright in the hole but not when it is lying on the ground after it has been removed (penalty 2 strokes).

I'll probably get criticism from many golfing corners on this short introduction to the main rules, and on what I've excluded, but as a qualified and experienced PGA pro and PGA Rules Referee and Tournament Administrator who's run countless Rules and Etiquette courses in Switzerland for new golfers, I know what you need to get started. Your first experiences on the golf course will not be in competition format. Get curious, though. Find out the rulings for situations I haven't covered here. Learning by doing is always more powerful than trying to learn from textbooks. Etiquette from day one; rules as you go.

Rules & Etiquette HIIT

- Re-read the Etiquette section of this chapter every night before you go to bed for one week!

- If you can't sleep after that, get yourself a copy of the rules book. Sweet dreams!

Golden nuggets

Etiquette:

- Respect your fellow golfers
- Respect the golf course
- Pace of play – No faffing!

Rules:

- Get acquainted with the most-often-occurring rules situations
- Ask about other situations as and when they occur

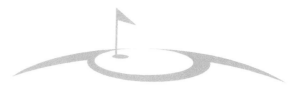

CHAPTER 10

Full Swing Progression

'I'm enjoying this – I can hit it! But how do I get better?'

I worked as the head pro at Panmure Golf Club in Angus next to the brutal Open Championship Links at Carnoustie from 1992 to 1995. As I drove to work each morning from Monifieth to Panmure, I would often pass the lone figure of Liz McColgan running along the road. No entourage, no trainer, no running partners. They probably couldn't have kept pace with her, anyway. Liz is one of the most successful female British middle- and long-distance track and road running athletes – twice 10,000 m Commonwealth Games gold medallist in 1986 and 1990, Olympic Games silver medallist in 1988, World Championships gold medallist in 1991, and winner of the New York Marathon (1991), Tokyo Marathon (1992) and London Marathon (1996). At that time, I gave lessons to someone who had encouraged her to join her local athletics club, the Hawkhill Harriers, at the age of twelve. I will never forget him telling me that although she wasn't the most talented runner (as she admits herself),[24] her attitude and application for the sport were extraordinary. Her record is testament to her powerful mindset, focus and determination as much as to her physical prowess.

Dr Dave Alred writes in his inspiring book *The Pressure Principle*,[25] the attributes you need to improve in anything, in this very deliberate order, are:

1. Attitude

2. Application

3. Ability

I've taught many golfing 'Liz McColgans'. No label of actual or perceived talent should be put on anyone at the start of any new endeavour; it's number 3 on the list. Put in the effort and commitment, and let's have fun and see what the outcome is. No limits mentality.

So how are you getting on? You've made it to Chapter 10 and hopefully your golf swing has some solid fundamentals installed: club swing direction, posture, grip and rhythm. You will have improved your coordination to the ball through practice, even if there is little consistency as yet. And when you do connect with the ball, it should be going a good distance. Great. Now we need to go into a little more detail.

Before we do so, I want to thank my coach for the past two years, Jean-Jacques Rivet, for his part in my development as a player and as a coach. He is an amazing font of knowledge and experience and a true gentleman. I am indebted to him for some of the wisdom and coaching in the following paragraphs.

All the following tips are geared towards either improvement in strike, consistency of strike or directional control; so, before I start, let me give you a simplified version of ball flight mechanics so you can understand why the ball goes where it goes and help you identify what you need to adapt (see Figure 20).

Figure 20 (top) gives the terminology for the different ball flights for a right-hander. In Figure 20 (middle), the ball starts where the clubface is aiming at impact – closed starts left, square starts straight and open starts right. And in Figure 20 (bottom), the spin on the ball is affected by the clubhead swing direction relative to your ball-to-target line – out-to-in gives right spin, in-to-square-to-in goes straight, in-to-out gives left spin.

Figure 20

*Ball flights
for the right-
handed golfer*

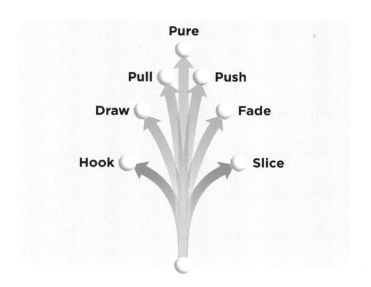

Club face angle
at impact

Swing path
through the ball

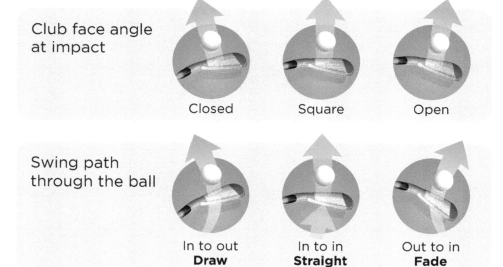

Address position adaptations

Grip: top-hand fine-tuning, linking the hands and pressure

In Chapter 3, I taught you the baseball or 10-finger grip. What is most important for your grip is the natural position of your top hand. A double check and fine-tuning for the top-hand position is to take a practice swing, stop at the top of the swing, take away your bottom hand and swing the club down and through with the top hand only. If this is uncomfortable or doesn't feel powerful, then your top hand needs to sit a little more on top of the grip (see Figure 21). Repeat the above process as necessary until you find your most powerful 'throwing' position.

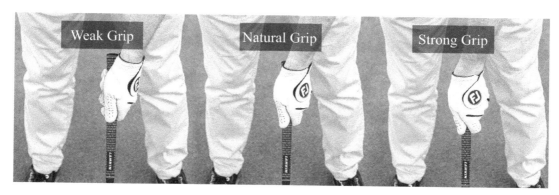

Figure 21 *Left hand grip variations*

The baseball grip has its limitations: with no linkage between the top and bottom hands, the coordination of left and right side is not optimal. In addition, the hinging or leverage of the trail arm is not as effective as in other grip positions. For these reasons, you will usually only see beginners, juniors or people with small hands using it. Experiment with the two most popular grip positions: the interlock grip and the overlap grip (see Figure 22). Neither have the drawbacks of the baseball grip.

Use whichever grip feels most comfortable to you. At the start, you will probably grip the club too tightly, which, as mentioned in Chapter 3, we want to avoid. As the grip becomes more comfortable, try and get back to a constant and lighter grip pressure.

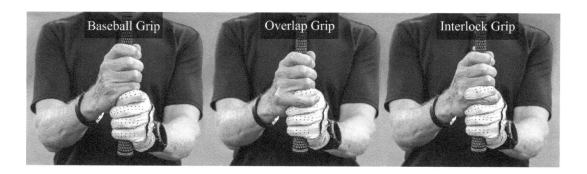

Figure 22 *Overlap and interlock grip*

Grip: direction influences

Wherever the clubface is facing at impact is where the ball starts (see Figure 20/ middle). The grip has the biggest influence on this position. For the sake of simplicity, I'll explain this for the right-hander (sorry, lefties – just think in opposites).

If the left hand is in its natural position (see Figure 21) or slightly more on top of the grip, the clubface has a good chance of returning to square at strike. If the left hand is too far on top of the grip or in a so-called 'strong' position, the left forearm will over-rotate through strike, tending to shut (point left) the clubface at strike and sending the ball left, albeit powerfully. If the left hand is too far under the grip at address (disaster position!), the left forearm will counterrotate through strike, opening (pointing right) the clubface and sending the ball right. Avoid this grip position at all costs. I have *never, ever, ever,* seen a good, powerful golf swing coming from a weak top-hand position. It causes all sorts of contortions of the wrists, arms and body in an attempt to close down an open clubface. Horrible! That's why I often say to my students 'I love left' (ie the ball going left); it's powerful with potential and just needs a little adjustment.

As I mentioned in Chapter 3, the right hand is not quite in its natural position – it sits a little more on the side of the club than the left hand to get a good fit between the fold in the middle of the right hand (lifeline) and the left thumb so that, through impact, the leverage in the right elbow and wrist is more powerful. The interlock or overlap grip should give you a better fit than the baseball grip. Although the right hand has less directional influence than the left, a weak position where the hand sits too far on top of the left thumb will tend to open the clubface and a strong position will tend to shut the clubface.

For reference, look at tour players' grip positions. They are not all the same. The 'strong' grippers (left hand more on top) tend to be the long hitters as this position causes a lot of arm rotation and therefore speed through strike (akin to a powerful backhand in tennis), and they need a powerful lateral movement and body rotation to stop the clubface shutting too early. Great for power; however, they can also be wild off the tee if their timing is not good. It's unusual to find a straight, long hitter; watch some long driving tournaments – these players can hit the ball over 350 m but also into different zip codes!

Foot position adaptations

If there is one thing I've learned from teaching thousands of people in the last 30 years, it's that nobody moves the same way. That's why I don't teach a swing method (ie the same movements and positions for everybody regardless of body characteristics). Variances in joint mobility and muscle flexibility are the main factors causing differences in movement, and if these are limiting for you, **exercise!** Re-read Chapter 8; I encourage you to exercise regularly for longevity and *joie de vivre*. My preferences would be yoga or Pilates.

Experiment with your feet position at address. For simplicity, once again I'll explain for the right-hander. You may have noticed that in a powerful throwing motion and golf swing the pelvis rotation on the backswing is about half of the rotation of the forward swing: roughly 45 degrees versus 90 degrees. (Don't fret about these numbers. They are just a rough guide to give you a picture of good movement.) The positioning of the feet can have an enormous influence on this rotation. If I point both feet straight ahead, there's a good chance I'll be able to make a 45-degree pelvis turn on the backswing but will have difficulty turning 90 degrees on the through swing; therefore, turning the left foot out a little towards the target will help your mobility on the follow-through. This increased rotation can affect a more powerful body rotation. Think of the feet as the hands of a clock, so in the standard position the right foot points to 12 o'clock and the left foot to 11 o'clock. However, the further you turn that left foot towards the target, the more difficult it is to get a good backswing rotation. Equally, turning the right foot to the right will aid mobility on the backswing and hinder mobility on the downswing.

You have to experiment to see where you get your best movement. If a short turn on the backswing is your problem, turn the right foot out a little. If you are not facing your target in the finish position, turn the left foot out a bit more. Where I know the student has hip mobility limitations, I encourage a narrow stance and 'Charlie Chaplin' foot position or '10 to 2'. No rights and wrongs here, so just have some fun and find out what works and what doesn't.

Ball position

This also varies from person to person depending on mobility and flexibility. I recommend doing the 'hit the line' exercise from Chapter 3 often, varying where the line is from aligned with the mid-point between your feet to your front foot to find out where you get the most consistency. This will help identify your low point.

Ball position can also influence directional control. If you've got the hang of the swing direction from Chapter 3, the clubhead should be following your body and arms in a curving motion through strike. Think of the putting drill against the wall from Chapter 6 – you want the clubhead to strike the ball at the apex of the curve to send the ball straight ahead. Too early and the ball will start right of target, too late and the ball will start left of target (for the right-hander). Once again, experiment, watch what the ball flight does, relate it to Figure 20 and adapt as necessary.

That's your address position variables. You'll have noticed I never mentioned adaptation of posture. Stick to Chapter 3 description; that is your 'bread and butter' position. Get it natural and athletic, and don't change it.

Now for some more swing control – primarily for better and more consistent ball striking, although it will also have a positive influence on your directional control.

Swing adaptations

I am going to explain this in two parts: backswing and downswing. It's a logical and simple way to explain it, though it doesn't accurately reflect what happens. The golf swing is in continuous motion – fluidity is key to power. If you've learned the club 'throwing' motion and club direction – upright to flat to around – as described in Chapter 3, then you may already have a lot of what I shall mention here in place. There is method in my madness, but I want you to be able to know your swing, create awareness of your movement and be able to self-analyse. The golf swing is a complex movement and will get too complex and unnatural if you listen too much to (mostly) well-meaning advice. My intention is to give you more stability through efficient movement. This efficiency will translate into more consistency of strike and more speed in the clubhead as all the components that create speed in a golf swing – ground forces, body rotation, arm rotation and leverage, and sequencing – will work in harmony. The idea is also to reduce, not increase, the number of moving parts which will help simplify the movement and, therefore, make it more repeatable. So, let's crack on with some fine-tuning.

Backswing

Rotating the upper torso around the spine

The description is not reality – the spine will rotate with you and have some lateral movement – but picture turning around the spine as the axis. The first image from Figure 23 shows you the upper torso (not just shoulder) rotation in a completely upright position. This is what you are trying to repeat in the golf swing. Looks and feels easy, right? But it's more difficult to do in your golfing posture and with a club in your hands. Try doing the full Figure 23 sequence – upright rotation, golf posture rotation, golf posture rotation with club. This does several things:

- **Consistency:** It stabilises the body position relative to the ball so you don't have to rely on the eyes as much to get the clubhead back to the ball.

- **Power 1:** By turning the upper torso and not just swinging the hands and arms back, you are creating potential energy to release, through the arms and clubhead, at the ball.

- **Power 2:** It creates coil – winding up the upper body, which will pull the pelvis with you and create a resistance against the ground – winding you up like a spring to later release that energy at the ball.

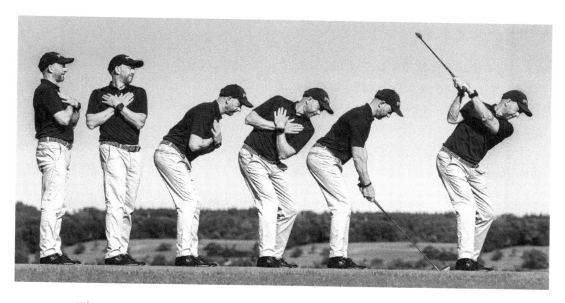

Figure 23 *Upper-body backswing rotation sequence*

I often see poor movement in which the rotation is not perpendicular to the spine. That makes it difficult to stay stable and balanced, doesn't wind up the 'spring' and can be dangerous for the back, particularly in causing slipped discs. Your rotation is critical, so check it often in the mirror or on video. How mobile you are will dictate how far you can coil. No need to reach a 90-degree shoulder position – go easy, stay stable, experiment with the foot positions in the previous section, and feel the spring winding up a little. The feedback you are looking for is tension in your gluteus maximus (your butt), inner thigh and maybe a little in your stomach muscles.

Lower back leg 'in concrete'

It's impossible to keep the upper body stable if the lower body is not. What you have already built in your address posture is helpful but not a guarantee of lower-half stability. The key is the lower back leg (right leg for right-handers, left leg for left-handers). You want to feel as though that lower leg up to your knee, is in concrete on the backswing – the whole sole of your foot flat on the ground and the lower leg remaining at right angles to the ground. This will ensure that the weight moves gradually to your back foot on the backswing and ideally into the heel, loading you up for a powerful forward motion.

Shoulder blades together, hands and arms passive

You may read or hear a lot about swing plane. It's not a concept I will cover here as, in my experience, it creates more confusion than clarity. If the body is moving as described in the previous backswing paragraphs and you keep your hands and arms passive, particularly in the first phase of the backswing (up to hip height), then you will be swinging on 'your plane'. This depends largely on your mobility and flexibility. I recommend keeping the distance between your shoulder blades the same as it is at address during the whole swing but particularly in the 'takeaway' – from start to hip height. This keeps the upper arms connected to the body so that the upper-body rotation dictates where the hands and arms, and ultimately the club, swing. You should then see the clubhead remaining 'outside' the hands up to hip height (see

Figure 5 in Chapter 3). As the rotation continues, the trail arm (right arm for right-handers) will naturally start to bend as the right shoulder comes closer to the club than the left shoulder. Get the hinging of your trail arm and wrist – two powerful levers in the golf swing – by gripping the club lightly and letting the weight of the club create the leverage naturally. This also prevents any unnecessary manipulation – opening or closing – of the clubhead. It's not the only way, but it's the easy way.

That's how you get a great backswing – with all the potential power created, and stability and clubface control to boot.

Downswing

Refer to the swing sequence images in Figure 5 (from Chapter 3) to help you visualise the following explanations.

I'm often asked, 'How should I start the downswing?' Well, if you've completed the backswing successfully, as described in the preceding paragraphs, you will already have started the downswing. The 'spring' that you have wound up will not want to stay wound up. It's not comfortable to hang on to the tension; it will want to release from the ground up – as in the throwing motion. Remember I said there was method in my madness at the beginning of the 'Swing adaptations' section? Your weight will already be shifting to the front foot, which in turn will push into the ground to stabilise the body (otherwise, you'll fall over – something the body never wants to do). This will create a rotation of the pelvis, then the upper body, and then translate it into arm speed and ultimately clubhead speed... if – and this is a massive if – you haven't completely screwed up this natural sequence by tensing up your shoulders, hands and arms in an attempt to hit the ball as hard as you can. The secret to power is in the sequencing, not in the upper-body strength, so I'm only going to mention two things to be aware of in the downswing.

Pressure in the ground – right heel to left toes (right-hander) for as long as you can

I had a strange dream a few months ago. Not unusual for me, as some of my close friends will testify, but nonetheless quite remarkable. John Daly, a famous PGA Tour pro and one of golf's more colourful characters, was giving me tips: 'Turn your right foot out a bit, Andrew, and try and kick the ball with the inside of your right foot on the downswing'. When I woke up, I thought, 'Right foot turned out a bit makes sense as I know I have a slight mobility problem in my right hip but kick the ball!?' Then I thought about the body and weight positions you need to kick a football with the instep of your right foot, and I realised dream-John's advice was perfect. The body is in a 'closed' position to the target (aiming right), allowing the club to swing beautifully from inside the target line – perfect throwing motion. In addition, the weight is in the left toes and right heel – perfect ground forces. What a great picture! I later found out from my learned colleague, Russell Warner, that this is already known as sound biomechanical golf movement. I'd never heard of it before, so thanks to my subconscious and Mr Daly for bringing this picture to my attention.

As the 'spring' pulls you onto the left side, imagine getting into position to kick the ball with your right instep. This will prevent the common tendency to 'hit from the top' or overuse the shoulders, arms and hands to 'muscle one out there'.

Allow the arms and club to swing straight down

If you have coiled properly on the backswing, you have created space in front of your chest to swing the arms and club back down into. The reason I use the word 'allow' is that if the grip pressure is not too tight, gravity will help you 'drop' the hands, arms and club down in front of you. The club should be in almost a right-angled relationship to your spine halfway back down to the ball. Welcome back to the efficient 'throw'/baseball/tennis position from Chapter 3. This is not a position to 'try' to get into; it should be a natural consequence of what has happened before and being mentally 'ready to let go of the club and propel it forwards'. Easy to say, but at this stage your brain is telling you to 'hit the ball' not 'swing and release the club'. Here is the massive 'if' that I mentioned earlier in this section: if your hands, arms and shoulders are relaxed, you are in a position to swing and release. If there is tension, it disrupts the sequence – ie we start from the arms and upper body instead of from the ground up. So, how do you relax? Back to Chapter 3: grip pressure, breathing, centring, mouth open and relaxed, or whatever works for you. This is how you get rhythm, and rhythm is sequencing the movement.

I often tell my students to picture starting in the address position with your hands against a table. The goal of the hands and arms swing is to get the hands back under the table at strike. A common error is to swing the hands down on top of the table and not under the table; then, the 'penny drops' about 'allowing the hands and arms to swing straight down'. Check out my video 'Hands under the table' from the accompanying video series.

Golden nuggets

Some tips and tricks to try out (reference Chapter 10 on Golf Yourself to Life Series – code at back of book):

- Hit the line
- Constant grip pressure
- Aim low/inside at the ball
- Bad swing and good swing
- Eyes-shut practice swings
- Blow the ball

- Kick the ball with your instep

- RH index finger and thumb off

- Left arm behind left shoulder joint to strike

- Heavy arms

We all want to hit great shots. It's fun, and bad shots suck! It's easy to get frustrated if you hit a lot of bad shots, but frustration doesn't help the learning process. If you become aware of what is causing the bad shot, through trial and error, you can solve the problem, improve the position, movement, feeling or thought, and move on. Learn from the poor shots. Accept that you are going to hit a lot of them, and pay attention to them to identify the problem and find solutions. That's how you'll improve and succeed. Stay patient, stay relaxed, get feedback and get curious. And if you need help with patience and relaxation, start meditating!

THE FINAL WORD

Nods to the past, vitality in the present, wallow in the future

My sincere hope is that you have reached the end of this book with some exciting experiences behind you. Shots that have flown high and far, approaches that have ended up close to the flag, bunker shots that have popped up easily out of the sand, and putts that never looked like missing before disappearing into our ultimate destination – the hole. I would also be surprised if you haven't experienced days when you thought you'd turned up to the range in somebody else's body and when nothing you tried seemed to get you the desired result. Unfortunately, the more complex a movement is, the more difficult it is to repeat. Complexity is the challenge of this sport; that's why my endeavour as a coach is always to keep the number of moving parts to a minimum and keep the thought process as simple as possible. As long as there is a balance of success, failure and learning, then you will progress.

Despite some recurring frustrations, I hope you have also started to appreciate what an amazing game this is; the varied locations, landscapes, flora and fauna. The community of golfers who have made this sport part of their lifestyle and friend circle. The health benefits of being in wide open, green spaces, walking up to 10 km in 4 hours, switching off from work or social stresses, feeding the brain with fresh new challenges every few minutes, and immersing yourself in your surroundings with family, friends, colleagues, strangers or on your own. The knowledge that golf is a sport you can enjoy long after you've hung up your football boots, tennis shorts or running shoes. And above all, the fun it can bring. As I mentioned at the start of this book, life is supposed to be fun!

In her book *The Power of Meaning*, Emily Esfahani Smith identifies four pillars that give life meaning:[26]

1. Belonging

2. Purpose

3. Storytelling

4. Transcendence

For me, and many of the sixty million other people worldwide who play golf, this great game delivers on all four:

1. A sense of belonging to a group of like-minded individuals in a community or club.

2. A purpose to get dressed up and prepared for, to gain new and fulfilling life experiences.

3. Telling stories of situations, places, successes, failures and comic occurrences from our golfing experiences all over the world. What's a story if there is no-one to tell it to? The golfing community will want to hear you.

4. Transcending the physics of propelling a ball from one point to another by training your body and mind to work in harmony and allowing them to perform extraordinary tasks without conscious thought.

You are amazing when you allow yourself to be, and golf can help you live a meaningful life. I wish you a long, healthy and abundant time on this wonderful planet, and may you get more out of it by golfing yourself to life!

AFTERWORD

This book and accompanying online material deliberately adopt a 'do-it-yourself' approach to getting you started in golf. As a coach, I also offer a 'do-it-with-you' approach for those who desire feedback from a trained eye. I offer these services both online and 1-on-1. To find out about my coaching packages to accelerate your progress from beginner to handicap golfer, check out my website golfyourselftolife.com. It would give me great pleasure to help you advance and get more enjoyment from this brilliant game.

Nature is integral to golf. By purchasing this book, you have also made a contribution to enhancing nature in golfing environments and promoting a culture of sustainable management in golf. To see how your contribution is being used, check out the golfyourselftolife.com website. Many thanks for your support.

ENDNOTES

1. This is the motto of Abraham-Hicks Publications.

2. Michael Anthony, *How To Be Happy* (2011), www.amazon.co.uk/How-Happy-Have-Changing-World-ebook/dp/B005U26JJE, accessed 5 October 2021

3. A golf handicap is a numerical measure of a golfer's potential that lets players of varying abilities compete against one another. It is calculated by playing against the par (pro average result) of the golf course – a sum of the individual pars for each of the 18 holes. The handicap tells you how many more strokes, on average, you would take than a professional player; for example, a player taking 80 shots on a par-70 golf course has played to a handicap of 10. Better players have lower handicaps.

4. Renée Mauborgne/Blue Ocean Strategy and Colin Weston, 'Creating new golf markets that make the competition irrelevant', The ModGolf Podcast (18 April 2019), modgolf.fireside. fm/062-renee-mauborgne

5. Edwin Roald, '7 Health Benefits of Golf – Why golf is good for mind and body', EIGCA (18 January 2016), www.eigca.org/Articles/21696/7-health-benefits-of-golf-why-golf-is-good-for-body-and-mind, accessed 15 October 2021

6. World Health Organization (WHO), 'Cardiovascular diseases (CVDs)', 11 June 2021, www.who.int/news-room/fact-sheets/detail/cardiovascular-diseases-(cvds), accessed 12 October 2021

7. www.golfandhealth.org/mental-health, accessed 15 October 2021; Dr A Murray, L Daines, D Archibald, R Hawkes, L Grant, N Mutrie, 'The relationship and effects of golf on physical and mental health: a scoping review protocol', *British Journal of Sports Medicine*, 50/11 (no date), https://bjsm.bmj.com/content/50/11/647, accessed 15 October 2021

8. S F Yeager, R Heim, J Seiler, H Lofton, 'Self Monitoring – the way to successful weight management', Obesity Action Coalition (Winter 2008), www.obesityaction.org/community/article-library/self-monitoring-the-way-to-successful-weight-management, accessed 19 October 2021; R&A (Royal and Ancient), 'Golf and Health 2016-2020' (no date), https://tinyurl.com/4u9unekp, accessed 19 October 2021

9. B Farahmand, G Broman, U de Faire, D Vågerö and A Ahlbom, Golf: a game of life and death – reduced mortality in Swedish golf players', *Scandinavian Journal of Medicine & Science* in Sports (28 May 2008), https://pubmed.ncbi.nlm.nih.gov/18510595, accessed 6 October 2021

10. BBC News, 'Playing golf gives "all round health benefits"' (6 October 2016), www.bbc.co.uk/news/uk-scotland-edinburgh-east-fife-37567254, accessed 19 October 2021

11. CaddyTrek®, 'Right vs left-handed golf' (12 February 2019), https://caddytrek.com/right-vs-left-handed-golf, accessed 19 October 2021

12. This concept is mentioned in both Malcolm Gladwell's *Outliers* (Little, Brown and Company, 2008) and Daniel Coyle's The Talent Code (Random House Books, 2009)

13. J Kaufman, *The First 20 Hours* (Penguin Books, 2013); J Kaufman, 'The first 20 hours – how to learn anything' (TED Talk, 14 March 2013), https://tinyurl.com/4ujmmndk, accessed 9 October 2021

14. Daniel Coyle, *The Talent Code* (Random House Books, 2009)

15. Golf World Archive, 'Seve Ballesteros' Best Shots' with Former Caddie Billy Foster (2016), www.youtube.com/watch?v=OrP5R3gFAgo, accessed 10 October 2021

16. Loran Smith, 'Remembering the great Doug Sanders', *Gwinnett Daily Post* (21 April 2020), gwinnettdailypost.com, accessed 18 September 2020

17. S Magness and B Stulberg, *Peak Performance* (Rodale Press Inc, 2017)

18. Jayne Storey, Golf International Articles 2009–2014 (free e-Book), chi-performance Golf, http://chi-performance.com/wp-content/uploads/2015/07/Jayne-Storey-Gi-2009-2014-Free-eBook.pdf, accessed 20 September 2020

19. Dr Joe Dispenza, *Breaking The Habit of Being Yourself: How to lose your mind and create a new one* (Hay House UK, 2012)

20. Oxford English Dictionary, Google Search

21. Yves C Ton-That, *Golf Etiquette Quick Reference: A golfer's guide to correct conduct* (Artigo Publishing International, 2014)

22. Book: *Golf Rules Quick Reference 2019: A Practical Guide for Use on the Course – For Stroke Play and Match Play*, Yves C. Ton-that (Artigo Pub. Intl. LLc, 2018); App: Expert Golf – iGolfrules, Yves C. Ton-That (Artigo Pub. Intl. LLc 2018)

23. R&A, *Official Guide to the Rules of Golf* (Octopus Publishing Group, 2019)

24. N Drysdale, 'Liz McColgan: How training runs in the streets of Dundee led to Seoul silver and Tokyo triumph', *The Courier* (6 August 2021), www.thecourier.co.uk/fp/past-times/2426137/liz-mccolgan-tokyo, accessed 15 October 2021

25. Dr Dave Alred, *The Pressure Principle: Handle Stress, Harness Energy, and Perform When It Counts* (Penguin Life, 2016)

26. Emily Esfahani Smith, *The Power of Meaning: The true route to happiness* (Rider, 2017)

BIBLIOGRAPHY

Adler, Jonathan, *Golf Psychology: When Positive Thinking Doesn't Work* (Jonathan Adler, 2013)

Alred, Dave, *The Pressure Principle* (Penguin Life, 2016)

Ballesteros, Severiano, *Natural Golf* (Stanley Paul, 1988)

Bergeron, Ben, *Chasing Excellence* (Lioncrest Publishing, 2017)

Bennett, M and Plummer, A, *The Stack and Tilt Swing* (Gotham Books, 2009)

Blancos, Homero, *Neuroscience and Your Golf Swing* (Pedro Perez, 2011)

Bradley, Nick, *The 7 Laws of the Golf Swing* (DK Publishing Inc, 2004)

Burchard, Brendon, *High Performance Habits* (Hay House Inc., 2017)

Clarke, D and Morris, K, *Golf – The Mind Factor* (Hodder and Stoughton, 2005)

Coyle, Daniel, *The Talent Code* (Random House Books, 2009)

Coyle, Daniel, *The Little Book of Talent* (Random House Business Books, 2012)

Dispenza, Joe, *Breaking the Habit of Being Yourself* (Hay House Inc, 2016)

Doig, David, *Mind for Sport, The Tool Book For Sports Psychology* (David Doig, 2012)

Dotz, T, Hoobyar, T, and Sanders, S, *NLP: The Essential Guide* (Harper Collins Publishers, 2018)

Esfahani Smith, Emily, *The Power of Meaning* (Rider, 2017)

Faldo, Nick, *A Swing for Life* (Weidenfeld and Nicolson, 1995)

Fitzgerald, Matt, *How Bad Do You Want It?* (Aurum Press, 2016)

Gallwey, W Timothy, *The Inner Game of Golf* (Jonathan Cape Ltd, 1981)

Herrigel, Eugen, *Zen in the Art of Archery* (General Press, 2011)

Hicks, Esther and Hicks, Jerry, *Ask and It Is Given* (Hay House Inc, 2018)

Kabat-Zinn, Jon, *Wherever You Go, There You Are* (Piatkus, 2000)

Kaufman, Josh, *The First 20 Hours* (Penguin UK, 2013)

Kelly, Homer, *The Golfing Machine* (Golfing Machine, 1969)

Lipton, Bruce H, *The Biology of Belief* (Hay House Inc, 2006)

Leadbetter, David, *The A Swing* (St Martin's Press, 2015)

Magness, S, and Stulberg, B, *Peak Performance* (Rodale, 2017)

Mumford, George, *The Mindful Athlete* (Parallax Press, 2016)

Nicklaus, Jack, *Golf My Way* (Pan Books, 1976)

Nilsson P, and Marriott, L, *Every Shot Must Have a Purpose* (Penguin, 2005)

Parent, Joseph, *Zen Golf: Mastering the Mental Game* (Doubleday, 2002)

Penick, Harvey, *Little Red Golf Book* (Simon and Schuster, 1992)

Rotella, Bob, *Golf Is Not A Game of Perfect* (Simon and Schuster, 1995)

Rotella, Bob, *How Champions Think* (Simon and Schuster, 2015)

Salzberg, Sharon, *Real Happiness: The Power of Meditation* (Workman Publishing, 2011)

Schonbrun, Zach, *The Performance Cortex* (Birlinn Ltd, 2018)

Shoemaker, Fred, *Extraordinary Golf* (Penguin, 1997)

Smalley, Susan, *Fully Present* (Lifelong Books, 2010)

Valiante, Gio, *Fearless Golf: Conquering the Mental Game* (Random House Group, 2013)

Watson, Tom, *Getting Up and Down* (Vintage Books, 1987)

Whitmore, Sir John, *Coaching for Performance* (Nicholas Brealey Publishing, 2017)

RECOMMENDED RESOURCES TO ASSIST LEARNING AND IMPROVEMENT

GOWOD – mobility first: www.gowod.app

BLACKROLL® – Fascia and Fitness: https://blackroll.com

Golf Coach App – Online golf coaching video analysis: https://golfcoachapp.com

Golf Yourself to Life – Video course: Go to www.golfyourselftolife.com and click on the call-to-action button, 'Video course accompanying book'. You will be directed to my Thinkific courses site. Click on, 'Golf Yourself to Life – video course'. At the payment page, use the following code to gain free access to the course: gytlbook

RECOMMENDED GOLF EQUIPMENT SUPPLIERS

Ping: ping.com

Callaway: callawaygolf.com

Golfbidder (new and second-hand equipment): golfbidder.co.uk

ACKNOWLEDGEMENTS

I must make reference, and pay homage, to the highly qualified and experienced golf coaches I have learned from, both in 1-on-1 coaching exchanges and at the many PGA education seminars and events that I have attended during my career. The following is a list, in no particular order, of those who have most significantly influenced my methodology and coaching delivery:

Jean-Jacques Rivet, Mike Bender, Mike Adams, Gary Smith, Martin Hall, James Leitz, Jonathan Wallett, Dr Christian Marquardt, John Jacobs, Russell Warner, Jimmy Murray, Scott Cranfield, Denis Pugh, John Garner and Brad Faxon. I thank you all for your wisdom.

I would also like to acknowledge those who have assisted and encouraged me to get my methodology down in writing, pictures and videos: Gila Sellam, Emanuel Stotzer, Erika Jakob, Eva Broz, Gabor and Christine Samogyi, Werner Loisch, Karin Jorga, Beat Herzog, Madeleine Regli, Leo Rupf, Luke Cullen, Peter and Rahel Schüpbach, Basil Schüpbach, Louis and Daniela Glatz, Dieter Meier, Konrad and Carola Wirz, Hans Roth and Peter Wetzer. Thank you all for your support.

THE AUTHOR

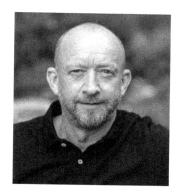

Andrew Cullen was born and brought up in Edinburgh, Scotland. He lived just five minutes' walk from the Royal Burgess Golfing Society, where he was a junior member and started the first year of his PGA apprenticeship.

In addition to his PGA qualification, he has an honours degree in Geography from the University of Glasgow, a Diploma in Sports Psychology from Newcastle College and is a PGA Qualified Rules Referee and Tournament Administrator.

He completed his PGA apprenticeship at the Bruntsfield Links Golfing Society, Edinburgh, in 1991 and gained his first head professional appointment in 1992 at Panmure Golf Club in Angus, Scotland. He developed his career further in Cornwall, England, as the head pro at Newquay GC, and later as Director of Golf at Roserrow G & CC. In 2003, he moved to Switzerland to become the head pro at Golf Club Limpachtal (2003–2008), Aetingen; he then became head pro at Golf Club Rheinfelden (2008–2015), and he is currently a freelance PGA professional working at Golf Club Markgräflerland in Kandern, Germany, and at a private indoor golf simulator studio in Basel, Switzerland.

Andrew still competes regularly on the Swiss PGA Seniors Tour and has one win to date at the 2015 Swiss PGA Tour at Golf & Country Club Basel in Hagenthal-le-Bas, France.

If you'd like to get in touch with Andrew, please use one of the following contact points:

🌐 www.golfyourselftolife.com

🌐 www.acgolf.ch

[f] Golf Yourself to Life

[in] Andrew Cullen

[○] golfyourselftolife

[YouTube] acgolf18

Lightning Source UK Ltd.
Milton Keynes UK
UKHW050740121221
395484UK00002B/3

9 781781 336519